Contents

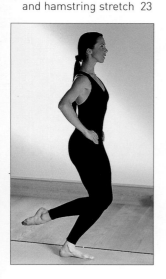

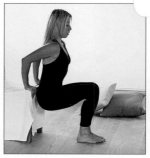

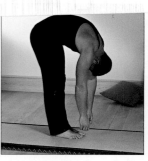

How to use the Pilates deck

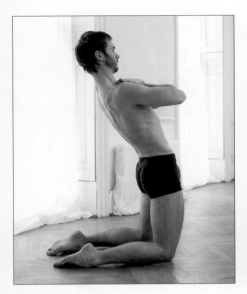

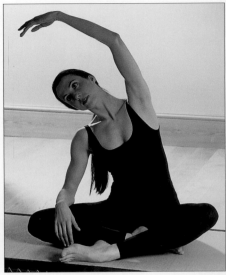

Above: The Back Bend, a core-strength exercise, in which the spine is lengthened.

Above: This side stretch relieves the body of tension, and liberates the spine and joints.

This pack is designed as an introduction to the key elements of Pilates and takes you through a comprehensive range of exercises, including some yoga-based exercises. The aim is to benefit everyone by helping you to integrate Pilates in to your daily life. The pack offers a selection of warming up and mobility exercises, which aim to loosen up all parts of the body, ending with relaxation. There are abdominal and back exercises; upper and lower body exercises; stretches; yoga-based core strength exercises; and advice on designing a short or longer programme that suits your particular lifestyle. There are FAQs and a short glossary with some key terms that are often used.

The cards
On the front of the cards, there are step-by-step pictures of each exercise and descriptions of how the movements should be carried out. An annotated picture of the exercise on the reverse of the card highlights important areas, provides tips, checkpoints for the different positions, and outlines the benefits of each exercise. Each card describes the target muscles, the purpose of the exercise and how many repetitions are needed.

Short and long programmes to suit different lifestyles are provided, with a list of exercises showing the time and repetitions for each one.

When you start your routine, wear comfortable clothes that allow you to stretch. Use a good, firm exercise mat with padding that will protect your spine. Don't have a heavy meal before starting exercise and try to keep well hydrated. Take time to relax at the end of each session.

Breathing

Breathing is something you do unconsciously, but when you are relaxed and calm your breathing pattern is different from when you are tense, anxious or negative. Here is a simple breath control strategy that you can practise at any time. Regulating your breathing will enhance your body awareness and control and make you feel calm and centred.

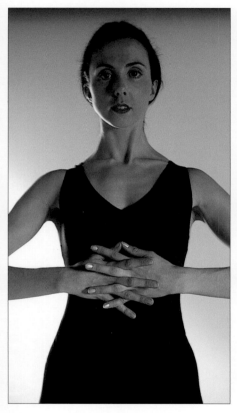 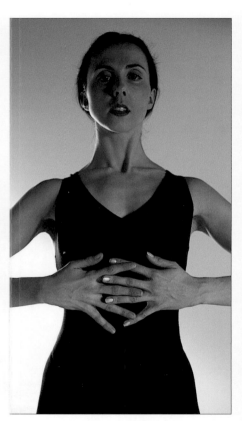

1 Place your hands with your palms under your chest, on your ribs, and your fingers loosely interlocked. Try to keep the shoulders relaxed. Inhale slowly and continuously through your nose, to a count of four. Do not strain, and do not hold your breath as this is the cause of tension in the muscles.

2 As you inhale, concentrate on allowing your ribs to expand laterally: your fingers should gently part. Don't let your ribs push upward and outward away from your spine, and do not arch the spine. Exhale slowly, expelling all the breath from your lungs, then repeat the breathing exercise.

Focus

When starting out on this or any other exercise programme, strive to master the general movement first, then focus on the breathing patterns. It is often the case that correct breathing patterns start to come naturally as the body tries to help itself, but you can practise breathing control exercises when you are not moving to help you learn the correct technique.

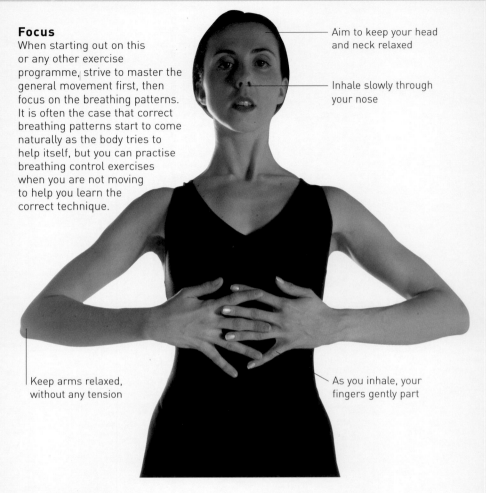

Aim to keep your head and neck relaxed

Inhale slowly through your nose

Keep arms relaxed, without any tension

As you inhale, your fingers gently part

Benefits

- If you learn to control your breathing while practising Pilates as well as during daily activity, it will help you to maintain your energy and stay relaxed and calm.
- Regulating breathing will enhance your body awareness and control and make you feel calm and centred. It can also calm your breathing pattern.

Breathing laterally

During breathing exercises be careful not to let the ribs flare up (push upward and outward away from your spine), which sometimes goes hand in hand with arching the spine. Aim to keep the ribs the same distance from your hips, just sliding them out to the sides and then back again as you breathe. This is described as 'breathing laterally'. This exercise may need to be repeated a few times until it comes naturally.

Building Core Strength

By stabilizing the torso you are creating a co-contraction between the abdominal muscles and the back muscles. This means that all these muscles are working together to create a stable entity.

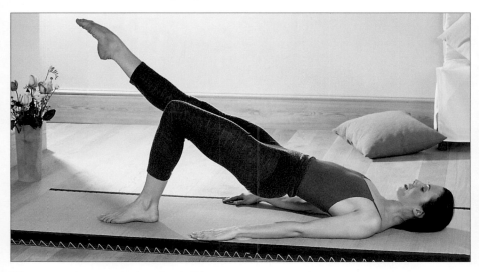

Pilates exercises are designed to build up your core strength.

Locating the transverse abdominis
Sit or stand upright, inhale and pull your stomach toward your back, imagining that you are trying to pull your tummy away from a waistband.

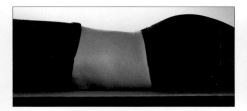

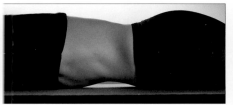

1 Lie on your tummy with your head relaxed and supported on your folded hands or on a small cushion under your forehead. Keep your head in alignment with your back and the back of your neck long, without shortening the front. Try to keep your hip bones on the floor and relax your shoulders.

2 Inhale, then, as you exhale, pull your navel toward your spine, trying to create an arch under your abdominals. You may not be able to lift very far up when you first try this movement: this is not important as long as you understand the concept. Gently lift your shoulders back and draw your shoulder blades down your spine.

4

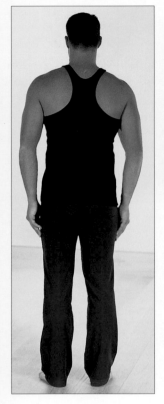

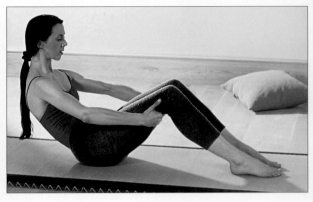

Every movement should be controlled via your abdominals. Keep bringing your attention and focus back to pulling your navel toward your spine. This is the basis of all of the Pilates exercises.

Benefits
• The stabilizing central muscles will be strengthened.
• You will be less prone to injury.

Abdominal muscles

The illustration displays the key abdominal muscles used in Pilates. These are the muscles used when we refer to 'working from a strong centre' or 'developing core strength.'

If sliding your shoulder blades down your spine seems like a baffling request, practise this subtle movement by standing up with your arms by your sides. Keeping your back straight, push your fingertips toward the floor. Do not force your arms down or lock them into position. Try to keep the shoulder blades close to the back of the ribcage. This is useful for limiting tension around the shoulders, which makes you pull your shoulders up to your ears.

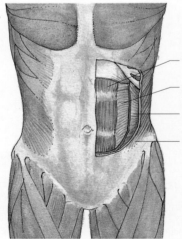

— rectus abdominis

— transverse abdominis

— internal abdominal obliques

— external abdominal obliques

Neutral Spine

The importance of neutral spine cannot be emphasized enough. It allows your spine to elongate and relax. Before starting an exercise, roll gently between the two extreme positions and then try to fall comfortably between the two.

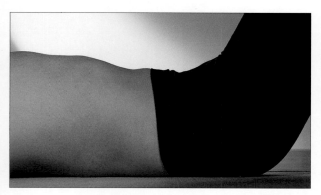

1 Tilt your pelvis, flattening your back in to the floor. If you suffer any pain while doing this, abandon the exercise and consult a physician before continuing.

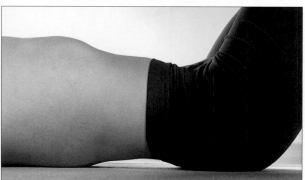

2 Tilt your pelvis in the opposite direction, creating an arch under your lower back. Make this movement slow and take care not to hold for too long or you may cause tension in your lower spine.

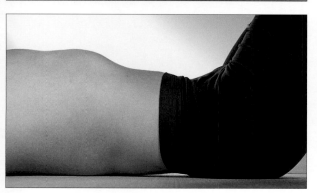

3 Find a position between these two extremes in which your back feels natural and comfortable: this is neutral spine. Unless otherwise stated, you should always work from this position during your Pilates routine.

KEY ELEMENTS OF PILATES

A healthy spine has natural curves that should be preserved and respected but not exaggerated. The term 'neutral spine' refers to the natural alignment of the spine. If you have any serious pain in your back, check with a physician before embarking on any exercise programme. Pilates is not intended to be an alternative to the prescription of a medical professional, but it can be a useful tool to accompany the recommendations of a specialist.

The main curves in the spine are in the following regions:

1 Cervical: the area behind the head, along the back of the neck, is concave; it should curve gently inward.

2 Thoracic: the largest area of the back curves very slightly outward.

3 Lumbar: the lower back should curve slightly inward; it should not be flat or over curved.

4 Sacral: the sacral curve is at the bottom of your spine and curves gently outward.

It is important to allow the spine to rest in its natural position to prevent stresses and imbalances. During Pilates movements you should ensure, unless otherwise directed, that your back is not flat or pushed into the floor, although this can be tempting in order to achieve a flatter tummy. What you tend to do in this position is grip at the hip flexors (the muscles located at the top of the thighs) thus creating tension in a place that is commonly tight anyway. You must also try to avoid curving your spine too much, as this pushes the abdominals forward and tightens muscles that are around the spine. Neutral spine lies in between these two extremes and echoes the natural and safe position that your spine prefers. Pilates exercises aim to help you achieve this position.

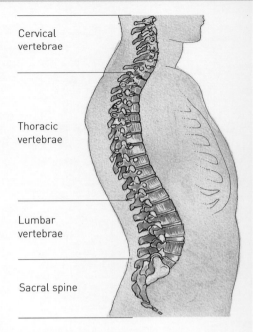

Cervical vertebrae

Thoracic vertebrae

Lumbar vertebrae

Sacral spine

The diagram shows the four natural spinal curves. These curves help to cushion some of the shock from our daily activities – even walking creates some mild stress. One of the key elements of Pilates is the close attention given to the alignment of the spine during all movements.

Benefits
- Stretching your spine in a controlled way during Pilates exercises can increase your range of movement, so that you have more freedom and mobility in your daily life.
- Stretching out the spine has been linked to a reduced rate of injury.
- A healthy, mobile spine will improve your mood; after a stretching session, many people have reported that they have greater flexibility, and feel refreshed and invigorated, with a general sense of wellbeing.

Posture

The body must be re-educated to cope with the stresses of daily life. In cases where the postural fault is severe, or there is pain, you should see a specialist before attempting this or any other exercise programme.

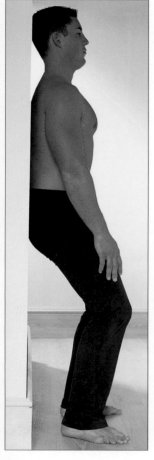

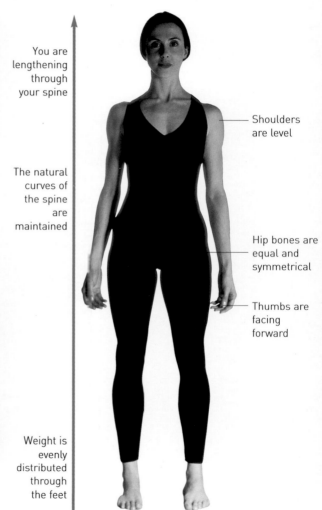

You are lengthening through your spine

The natural curves of the spine are maintained

Weight is evenly distributed through the feet

Shoulders are level

Hip bones are equal and symmetrical

Thumbs are facing forward

Once your core postural muscles have been strengthened, correct posture will become less of a muscular effort and much more of an unconscious act.

Stand in front of the mirror and carefully check your posture. Pay special attention to your hips, arms, shoulders, spine and weight distribution.

8

Key points
- Shoulders are level.
- Hip bones are equal and symmetrical.
- The thumb side of the hand faces forward.
- The knee joints are symmetrical and face forward.
- The ankle joints are symmetrical.
- The weight of the body is equally distributed between all four corners of the feet.
- You are lengthening through your spine.

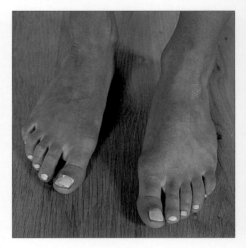

Benefits
- When your posture is correct, you will feel more positive and alert when you sit or stand upright.
- You will look lighter and slimmer and have a more toned appearance.
- The psychological effects are that you will feel more in control, confident and capable.
- You will feel healthier.

The weight of the body should be equally spread between all four 'corners' of the feet. Weakened muscles or rapid weight gain may have led the arches in the feet to collapse.

Pilates works by strengthening the key postural muscles, making it physically more comfortable to maintain the correct alignment.

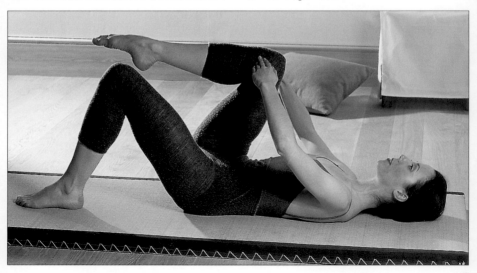

Arm Crosses

The movement should be continuous and flowing: think of the graceful way in which a ballet dancer's arms move. As you do the exercise, watch for tension in the neck; your spine should stay in neutral and your abdominals hollowed.

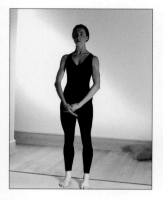

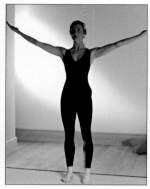

Benefits
- These are great for warming up the shoulders and upper back. Imagine you are trying to reach both sides of the room and lengthen out through your arms and up through your spine.
- The warm-up helps to get you in the mood for activity.
- The signals from your brain to your muscles are speeded up.

1 Stand and cross one hand in front of the other. Relax the shoulders, and lengthen through the spine.

2 Inhale and, as you exhale, take the arms to the sides. Slide the shoulder blades down the spine and lift arms.

Shoulder Circles

This movement is slow and controlled, breathing is wide and full through the ribs, the spine is kept in neutral, and the muscle core temperature is raised.

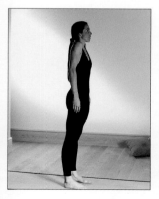

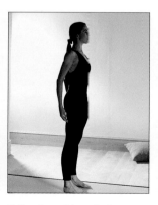

Benefits
- Relieves tension in the shoulders and upper back.
- Mobilizes the shoulders.
- Relieves tension in the shoulders and back.
- It is an easy, natural movement that many people stumble on when they are feeling stiff, and which can be done anytime.

1 Inhale. As you exhale, roll shoulders up to your ears.

2 Create as big a circle as you can one way then the other.

Arm Sweeps

As you perform this exercise, you will feel the tension draining away from your body. Try to keep the movement fluid and rhythmic and at a constant speed.

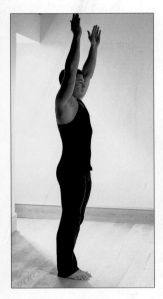
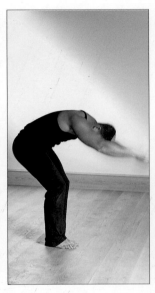
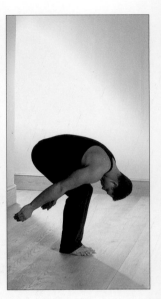

1 Stand with feet close together, knees and shoulders relaxed. Keep the abdominals hollowed. Extend arms overhead and lengthen up through the spine. Keep feet flat on the floor and head aligned.

2 Keep spine in neutral and adopt the correct breathing pattern. Inhale to prepare, then drop your chin to your chest and roll down through your spine, allowing your arms to begin to flow out behind you.

3 Bend your knees as your arms sweep back and again as you bring them forward and up over your head to begin again, lengthening up through your spine as you return to standing. Repeat five times.

Benefits
- This big, sweeping movement will wake you up and help with a fuzzy head.
- It also mobilizes the spine, lower body and the shoulders.
- Stretches spine.

Focus

The first part of any exercise routine should be a warm-up to raise the core temperature of your muscles. If you pull a cold elastic band too hard it snaps, but once it is warm it becomes more pliable and will stretch farther. The same applies to your muscles. The warm-up prepares you psychologically for activity, getting you in the mood. It also increases the efficiency of the neuromuscular pathways, thus speeding up the signals sent from the brain to your muscles. Keep your movements flowing and gentle during the warm-up: do not force your body or overstretch.

Rolling down the Spine

This is a really effective movement for mobilizing the spine, and can be refreshing if you have a stiff back. However, if you have problems with your spine take advice before trying this movement.

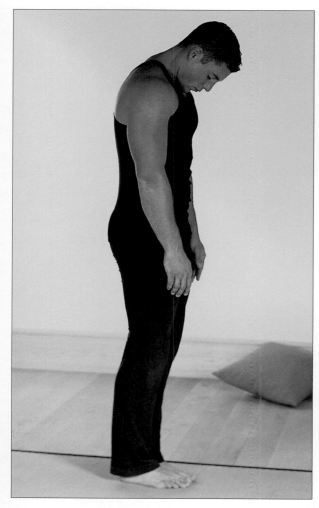

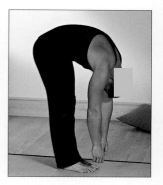

2 As you bend over from the hips, create a C-shape. Let the arms hang toward the floor. Feel the head relax and the shoulders drop. Don't sway backward or forward as you roll down.

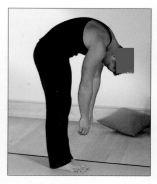

3 Start to curl back up, tilting the pelvis and trying to mobilize each part of the spine, uncurling it bone by bone and creating as much length as possible between the vertebrae.

1 Stand with your feet hip-width apart, balancing your weight evenly through your feet. Breathe in to begin and, as you exhale, lower your chin to your chest, and start to roll down toward the floor.

WARMING UP AND MOBILITY EXERCISES

Tips

- If you find it difficult, you can do it with bent knees or against a wall, and you can keep your hands on the thighs.
- Keep the movement flowing and remember not to collapse into it: the abdominals should not sag.
- Try not to lean backward or forward but keep your weight in alignment, with your feet flat on the floor. As you come up feel the crown of your head float up to the ceiling.

Purpose

To mobilize the spine and improve balance.

Target muscles

Designed to loosen/mobilize the spine.

Repetitions

Repeat 6 times.

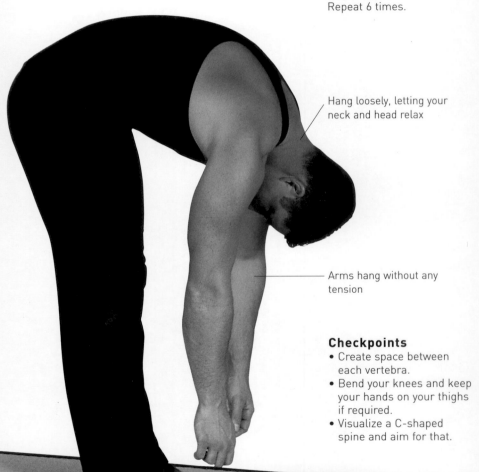

Hang loosely, letting your neck and head relax

Arms hang without any tension

Checkpoints

- Create space between each vertebra.
- Bend your knees and keep your hands on your thighs if required.
- Visualize a C-shaped spine and aim for that.

One Leg Circles

Circling the legs mobilizes the hip joints and also challenges core strength.
Because you aim to keep the hips still during movement of the lower body,
your thighs get a workout too. Keep the abdominals hollowed throughout.

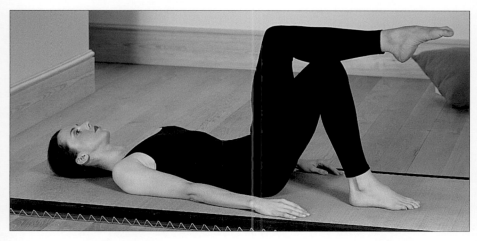

1 Lie on your back with your knees bent and your arms by your sides. Keeping your spine neutral, your head aligned and the supporting foot firmly on the floor, raise one bent leg. Ensure your hips are square and still. Then start to circle your knee. Make small circles initially, then larger ones, using your abdominals for control.

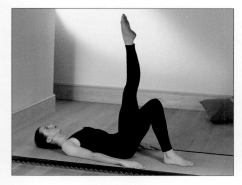

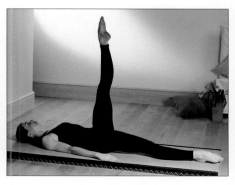

2 Straighten the moving leg; keep the other foot on the floor. Lengthen up through your toes to make your leg as long as possible. If your hips move, it would be better to work with a bent leg. Try to increase the size of the circle as you get stronger.

3 Straighten the supporting leg and lengthen. Continue to lengthen up through the circling leg. Make the circles as large as you can control. Do not try to progress to this position until you have control in the second position. Work from a strong centre.

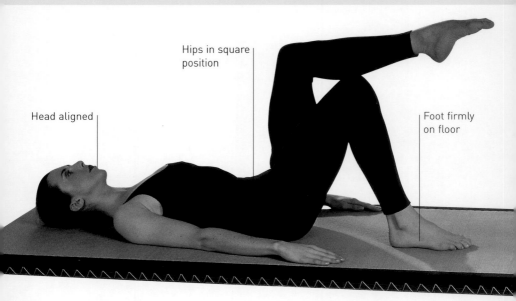

Hips in square position

Head aligned

Foot firmly on floor

Checkpoints for position 1
• Keep the hips square: don't let them lift from the mat.
• Keep the spine in neutral.
• Make the circle as large as you can control.

Checkpoints for position 2
• Keep the abdominals hollowed throughout the movement.
• Extend the circle as you grow stronger.

Checkpoints for position 3
• Try not to curve the spine too much.
• Lengthen through both legs.

Breathing and spine position
The breathing for this movement requires concentration: break each circle into semicircles, inhaling as your leg crosses your inner thigh and exhaling on the outer edge of the circle.

Make sure your spine stays in neutral and your shoulder blades glide down your back. The ribs may move away from the hips in this position so keep reminding

Benefits
• Increases mobility, which helps to keep the joints healthy and flexible.
• Challenges balance, strength and co-ordination.
• Helps to improve balance and mobilize the spine.
• Core strength is both challenged and improved.

yourself to control them. Make the circles flow and keep the movement continuous: think of a ballet dancer's grace and poise.

Purpose
To mobilize the hips and build core stability.

Target muscles
Adductors, hip flexors and abdominals.

Repetitions
Circle 5 times in each direction, then change legs and repeat.

The Shoulder Bridge

A very popular exercise in almost every class, this is a good mobilizer with which to start your session and a wonderful way to ease a stiff back. After this exercise your spine should feel loose and supple.

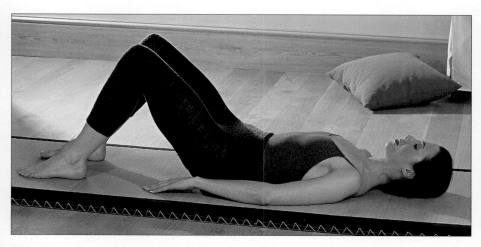

1 Lie on your back with your arms by your sides, slide your shoulder blades down your spine and lengthen your arms away. Bend your knees and place your feet hip-width apart flat on the mat. Your head is in alignment and your spine in neutral.

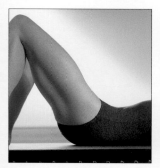 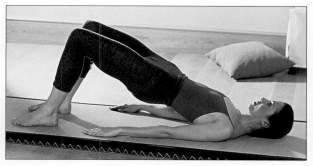

2 Tilt your pelvis and lengthen the tailbone away. The whole length of your spine should be in contact with the mat.

3 Slowly peel your spine up off the mat bone by bone, raising your hips toward the ceiling and keeping the abdominals flat and drawn down. In this position it is common to flare the ribs, so try to keep a constant distance between the hips and ribs. Make the movement smooth and flowing, inhaling as you lift and exhaling as you come down. Once you get used to the movement you can increase the stretch by taking your arms over your head.

WARMING UP AND MOBILITY EXERCISES

Target muscles
Erector spinae, abdominals.

Repetitions
Repeat 6 times.

Key benefits
- Mobilizes the spine and challenges the abdominals.
- Helps to keep joints flexible. Fluids are released into the joints, making the muscles more pliable, and reducing the risk of injury, as well as making muscular responses faster and more precise.
- Works abdominals and lower body.
- This exercise will help you to find your core strength.
- Your stamina and your energy levels will increase.
- This exercise can bring about a release of tension that will leave you feeling lighter and more relaxed.

Checkpoints
- Keep the hips level.
- Maintain the distance between the hips and the ribs.
- Make the movement flow.
- Aim to lift each bone in your spine off the mat in succession. You may find that, to begin with, your back lifts in two or three sections: try to create length between each vertebra.
- Use visualization: as you lower yourself to the floor, place each vertebra in turn on the mat, and imagine a pearl necklace sinking on to a velvet cloth.
- Keep hips perfectly level, and you should try to create as much distance between your hips and your shoulders as possible.
- Don't forget to tilt the pelvis as you begin the movement.
- To mobilize the spine fully, be sure to return to neutral as you lower your back to the floor, before you tilt the pelvis and start the next lift.

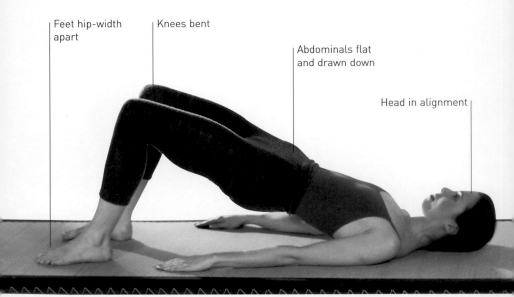

Feet hip-width apart

Knees bent

Abdominals flat and drawn down

Head in alignment

One Leg Circles

For this exercise, work at whichever level feels most comfortable.
Repeat five times in each direction then change legs. Lengthen up
through your leg and keep your spine in neutral.

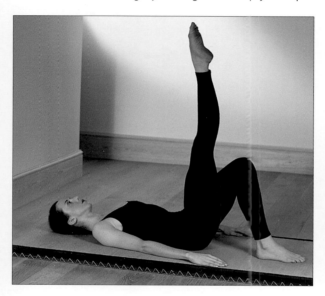

Lying on your back, circle
one leg, keeping your hips
very still. Start with small
circles then increase the
size of these, controlling
the movement with your
abdominal muscles.

Benefits
- This mobilizing Pilates
  movement helps to
  loosen the hip joint.
- Warms up the
  respiratory system
  (heart and lungs) as
  well as the muscles.
- Helps reduce the risk
  of injury.

Ankle Circles

This will give you a wonderful loose feeling in your ankles and really wake
them up. Repeat five times in each direction then change legs.

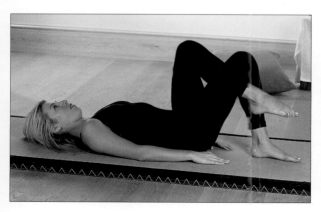

Lie in the same position
as for Knee Hinges, but for
this movement rest one leg
on the other. Slowly circle
your ankle in one direction,
then the other. Keep your
toes pointed and describe a
full circle. Concentrate on
the shape you are forming
and perform this movement
as slowly as you can bear.
Try to keep your spine in
neutral throughout the
entire movement.

Knee Hinges

Keep your spine in neutral and your abdominals strong throughout this movement. Relax your shoulders and neck. Repeat the exercise five times on each leg.

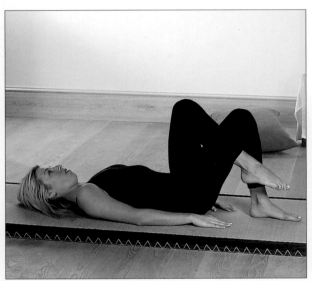

1 Lie on your back in the relaxation position. Lift one leg so that your thigh is at right-angles to the floor. Point your toe as you raise your foot.

Benefits
- The hinges mobilize the knees and warm up the ankles.
- The warm-up helps to set the mood for the rest of your workout.
- Prepares the body for cardiovascular exercise.
- Helps you to focus

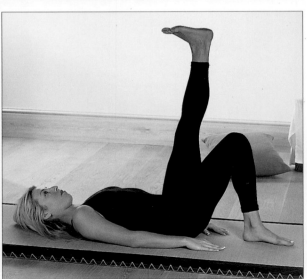

2 When the leg straightens flex your foot. Push your heel up toward the ceiling, then lower the foot. Think of your knee as a hinge, keeping the thigh still and limiting any movement in the hips. Exhale as you raise your leg, inhale as you lower it gradually to the floor.

Gluteals Stretch

You should not only tone the buttocks but also stretch the gluteals for best effect. Stretching lengthens the muscles and may help prevent injury. Stretch before and after cardiovascular exercise for optimum effect.

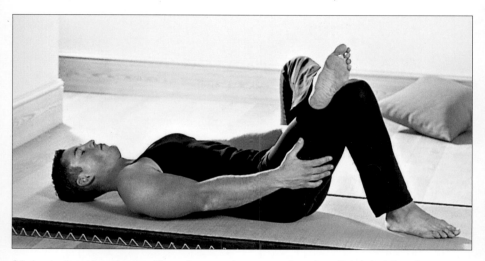

1 Lying in the relaxation position, place one leg across the other, lightly holding the supporting thigh with both of your hands.

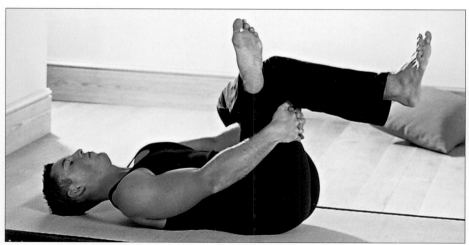

2 Exhale as you lift the supporting leg. Keep the abdominals strong throughout. Try to keep your neck and shoulders relaxed and do not overgrip.

20

Quadriceps Stretch

The fronts of the thighs tend to get quite tight because you use them for most lower body activities. If they get overtight they can cause knee problems. The main mistake people make with this exercise is to bend at the hip.

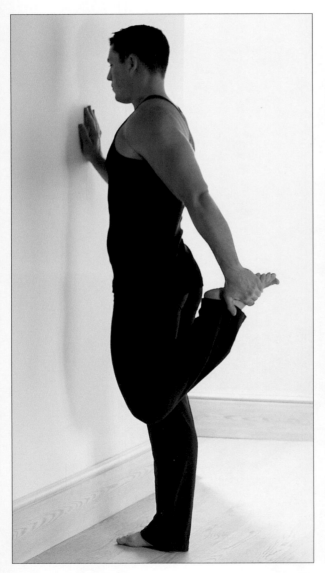

Stand facing a wall or other support. Bend one leg and raise your heel toward your bottom, keeping your knees in line with each other. Keep your abdominals hollowed. Exhale as you lift the leg. Watch for tension around the neck and shoulders, and keep your head in alignment.

Benefits
- Stretching affects your whole range of movement so that you have more freedom and mobility in your daily life and during sporting activities.
- Reduces the risk of injury.
- Gives a lift to the mood, leaving you feeling refreshed and invigorated, with a general sense of wellbeing.

Checkpoints
- Don't make the mistake of bending at the hip or you will lose the stretch. If you find it hard to hold your foot, loop a towel around it.
- Try timing your stretches because it is easy to rush them when tired.

Calf Stretch

The calf muscles can become quite tight, especially if you do much walking or climb a lot of stairs. This simple stretch is easy to do and will help to loosen up tight calf muscles.

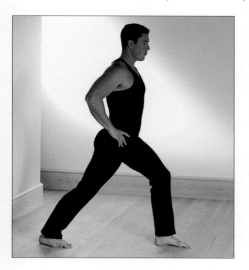

Standing up with your hands on your hips, take a big step forward. Keep your spine in neutral and lengthen up. Push your back heel in to the floor to feel a stretch in the back calf. During the movement, keep your abdominals hollowed and the head in alignment. If you cannot feel the stretch take a bigger step forward.

Checkpoints
- When you do this exercise, don't bounce, try to do the exercise smoothly.
- If you find the stretch uncomfortable, shorten the distance between your front foot and the back heel.
- If you have problems with your Achilles heel, don't do this stretch.

Adductor Stretch

This is a good stretch for the inner thighs. Stretching all the muscles in the legs helps to prevent knee and spine problems and reduces the risk of injury when exercising.

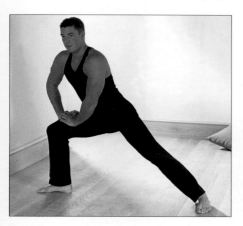

From standing, take a big step out to the side. Bend one leg so that the knee is over the heel and keep the other leg very straight. Don't collapse in to the stretch: watch the abdominals for sagging. Exhale gently as you stretch and feel the inner thigh lengthen.

Benefits
- Widens your range of mobility.
- Helps to induce a general feeling of wellbeing, and invigorates and refreshes.

Assisted Hip Flexor Stretch

This stretch uses a chair for support, but make sure it does not slip. It is particularly good for runners, but many other people also have tight hip flexors. You may feel the need to hold this stretch for longer than 30 seconds.

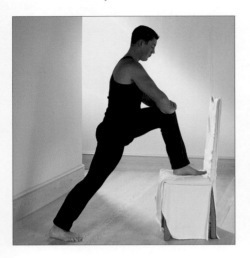

Stand up and rest one foot on a chair (or something lower). Bend the leg and lean in to the stretch on an exhalation, keeping your back heel on the floor. Keep your head in alignment, and your spine in neutral.

Benefits
• Mobilizes constricted muscles and induces a feeling of freedom.
• Prevents a tight lower back and weakened abdominal muscles.
• Helps to increase range of movement and thereby the flow of energy.
• Keeps the hip movement fluid so that you can move forward or backward.

Assisted Hamstring Stretch

This is another stretch that benefits from an additional support. The hamstrings tend to be tight in most people, and can cause back pain if left inflexible. If they do feel tight hold the stretch for slightly longer.

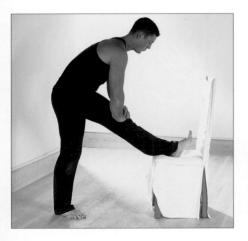

Standing on the floor, lift one leg and rest your foot on a support. Flex your foot and keep your leg straight, bending the supporting leg if this is more comfortable. Keep your head in alignment and your abdominals hollowed. Exhale as you ease in to the stretch. Support just above the knee and try not to push down on your leg.

Benefits
• Stretches the lower back and loosens the hamstrings, which stretch down the back of the thigh.
• Helps overall flexibility.

Drawing in the Abdominals

Whenever you get the chance, practise contracting your abdominals by drawing navel to spine. This action not only tones the abdominals but will get you used to the centring movement often used in Pilates exercises.

Take a few breaths and sit on a chair. Keep your back straight and your spine in neutral. Inhale and, imagining that you are wearing a tight pair of trousers, as you exhale pull your navel away from the waistband, making your waist smaller. Lengthen up through the spine.

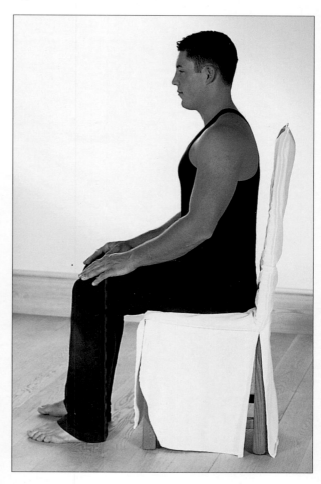

Benefits
- Helps the abdominals to become flatter, stronger and firmer.
- Aids correct alignment of body.
- Eases aches and stiffness.
- Quick and easy, so this exercise can be slotted in at any time during the day.
- With practise, will help to strengthen and lengthen the muscles that are needed to maintain good overall posture.
- The body will become rebalanced so that you will achieve optimum results during your Pilates sessions.
- Helps you to carry your body in the most efficient and safest way possible.

Action plan
You can do this simple exercise at home, at work or whenever you have a little time to spare. Try to pick a time when you feel fairly relaxed and not under pressure so you can really concentrate on the exercise and get the maximum benefit.

Wrist Circles

If you have been working on a computer it is helpful to give your wrists a stretch to make them feel looser. Remember to take a short break from your typing or writing every 20–30 minutes.

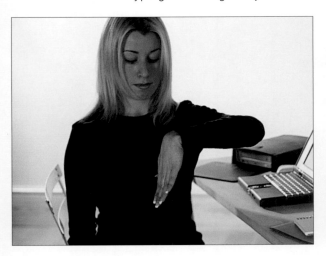

Start by circling your hand. Support it with the other hand at your wrist if this feels more comfortable. Circle in both directions, making a slow, full circle. Remember to keep the spine lengthened and the abdominals strong during the exercise.

Benefit
• Helps prevent RSI (repetitive strain injury) problems.

Hand Stretches

If you are working at a computer, writing or doing any other kind of repetitive movement with your hands during the day it can be beneficial to stop regularly and stretch out your hands.

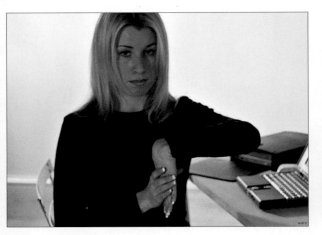

Keeping your hand straight and somewhat taut, draw your fingertips down toward the inside of your arm. Use the other hand to press them gently down. Now turn your hand in the other direction, drawing your fingernails toward the forearm.

Benefits
• Helps loosen wrists after repetitive work.

Drawing the Shoulder Blades Down

Standing or sitting, bring your arms to your sides with the thumbs facing forward. Slide your shoulder blades down your spine, keeping them close to the back of the ribcage so that they are not sticking out.

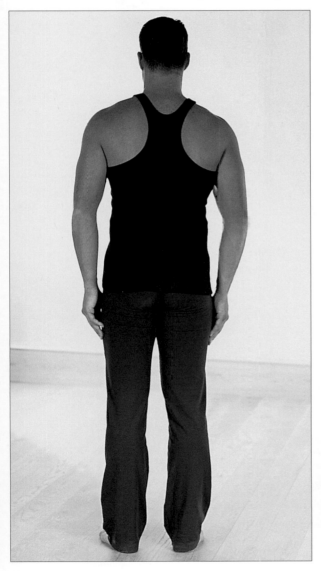

By gliding your shoulder blades down your spine, you will reduce the effect of any tension you are feeling in your neck and shoulders. Although hunching your shoulders up to your ears is a common reaction, it will exacerbate any discomfort you are already feeling in that area. Try to maintain the distance between your ear and shoulder at all times, unless otherwise stated. Throughout the day you can monitor the tension in your shoulders and try to become aware of situations that make them hunch up. For example, it is common for tension to increase when working at a computer for long periods of time, or when using the telephone, but by becoming aware of your habits and posture you can make a conscious and effective effort at reducing tension regularly through the day.

Benefits
- Relieves tension in the back and neck.
- The movement can be done regularly through the day to counteract tension caused by work practices.

Neck Stretch

When we sit for extended periods of time, especially while typing or writing, it is common to experience tension in the neck and shoulders. If you do store tension in your shoulders, these exercises may be helpful.

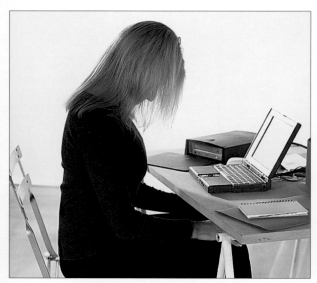

1 Keeping your spine in neutral and the abdominals strong, gently tip your head, letting your chin fall down toward your chest to feel a stretch in the back of your neck.

Benefits
- Stretches and mobilizes the muscles around the neck.
- If done regularly, eases tension and promotes relaxation.
- Makes you aware of correct posture to avoid neck pain.

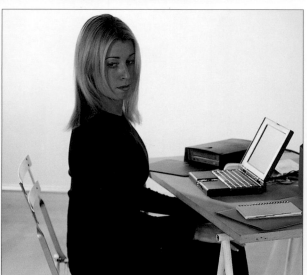

2 Turn your head slowly from side to side, taking care not to overstretch. Keep strong abdominals and a neutral spine.

Benefits
- Reduces stress and tension stored around the head.
- Relieves headaches.
- Maintains awareness of your body.
- Regular practice relieves pain in the neck area.
- Ensures that correct posture is maintained.

Walking Feet

Your feet and ankles can get stiff, and this exercise is designed to wake up the feet, ankles and calves.

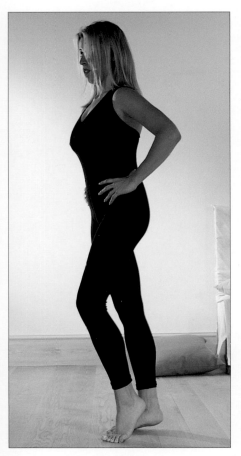

You need a strong, secure base for this exercise. From standing, lift the heel on one foot then the other in a natural walking movement, bending the knees. Keep the spine in neutral and the abdominals hollowed. Keep this movement rhythmic and continuous, always lengthening up through the spine.

Standing Balance

This is a more advanced way to warm up the feet and lower legs, which may also challenge your balance.

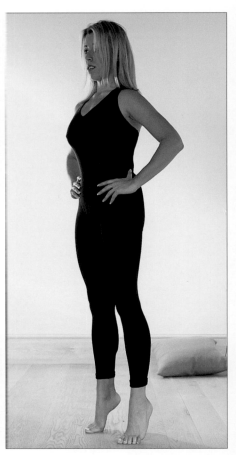

Stand with your feet hip-width apart and do not clench your toes, but relax. Keep your spine in neutral, abdominals hollowed, and place your hands on your hips to help you balance. Keeping your head in alignment, come up on to your toes. Hold for a few seconds, then lower your heels slowly to begin again.

Relaxation Position

This is not a movement, just a comfortable position. Try always to start and end your Pilates sessions with a couple of minutes in the relaxation position. It will help you to focus and also to get in contact with your body.

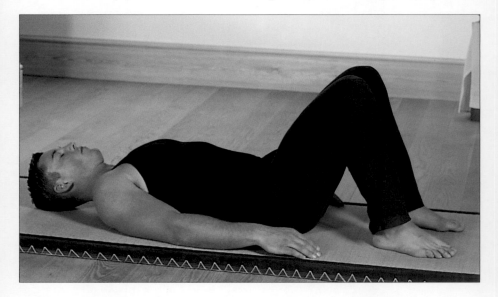

Lie on your back with your knees bent and your feet flat on the floor. Your spine should be in neutral. Relax your shoulders and let your shoulder blades gently glide down your spine, but do not force them into position. Your head should be in alignment with your spine and your arms relaxed by your sides. Breathe wide and full laterally, in through your nose and out through your mouth.

Checkpoints

- Take care not to create unnecessary tension; this would gradually create an imbalance in the body.
- Watch out for tension in the neck, jaw, shoulders and hips especially. However, tension can arise anywhere in the body, even in your feet, if you clench them.
- Check yourself all over for tension.

Benefits

- This simple position can be effectively used at any time during the day, whenever you get a chance to relax.
- Before moving on to postures, this relaxing warm-up primes the muscles, thus lessening the chance of injury.
- If you are tired, stressed or anxious, lying on the floor and connecting with it can allow your breath and emotions to calm down.
- Makes you feel relaxed and refreshed.
- Restores balance to the body.
- Regular relaxation provides benefits such as more refreshing sleep, more energy, extra alertness during waking hours and a general sense of wellbeing.

Rolling Back

Once you have mastered this movement, it can help to mobilize your back. However, you may find it quite difficult if your back has stiffened up – and make sure you work on a mat that gives you plenty of support.

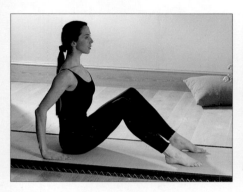

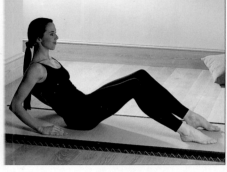

1 With your spine in neutral, knees bent and feet flat on the floor, place your hands near your hips with the fingers facing the feet. Inhale wide and full and draw the navel toward your spine. Lower your chin to your chest then use your hands for support and start to roll down to the floor.

2 Once you have rolled down as far as you can, exhale and, using your core strength, return to the starting position. Pull up through the crown of your head to create a long spine, then repeat. Use your arms only as support and avoid transferring all your weight on to your triceps.

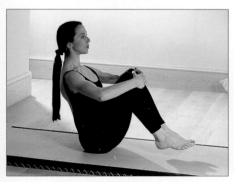

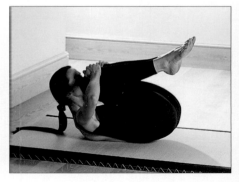

3 Sit upright with the spine in neutral. Lengthen up through the spine and imagine your head floating upward. Place the feet flat on the floor and hands just below your knees. Keep your elbows bent and the chest open. Take care not to tense or grip around your neck.

4 Inhale as you tilt the pelvis and curve the spine into a C-shape to roll back. Tuck in your chin and keep your thighs close to your chest. As you exhale, use the abdominals to pull you back up to the starting position. Try not to use momentum, but make the movement flow at a consistent speed.

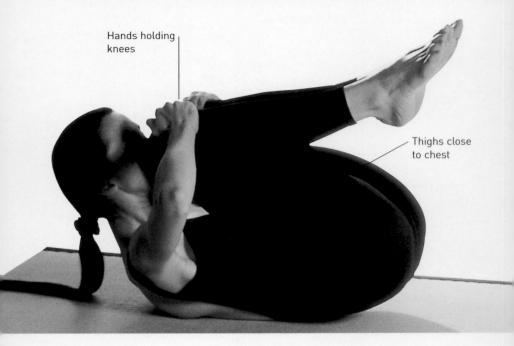

Hands holding knees

Thighs close to chest

Purpose
To mobilize and massage the back and strengthen the abdominals.

Target muscles
Erector spinae, abdominals.

Repetitions
Repeat 6 times.

Benefits
- The action of rolling carefully down each vertebra gently massages your spine and loosens it up.
- Your abdominals are exercised and strengthened when you pull them in while returning to the starting position.
- Your abdominals will become stronger, flatter and firmer.
- Your back will be free from stiffness.

Checkpoints
- Keep your feet flat on the floor for position 1.
- Lengthen up through the spine at the end of the movement.
- Tilt the pelvis.
- Keep the chin tucked in to the chest.
- Do not grip the neck.
- Use your abdominals to get you back to the starting position again.
- Try to place each vertebra on the floor, one by one. To do this, tilt your pelvis and curve your spine into a C-shape.
- Always use a mat that gives plenty of support to your spine.
- Use visualization when pulling in the abdominals. Imagine you are squeezing a sponge as hard as you can.
- Take care not to roll back on to your neck.
- Once you can roll down the spine with the hands on the floor, try rolling back; you may not roll back up on your first attempt.

The Roll-up

In spite of the name of this exercise, you begin by rolling down. It is an excellent way to strengthen the abdominals but is very challenging, so ensure you are comfortable and confident with the first position before moving on.

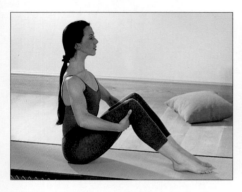

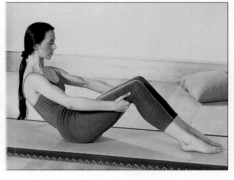

1 Sit upright with your feet flat on the floor and your knees bent. Hold the back of the thighs, with your elbows bent and your arms open; don't overgrip. Your spine should be in neutral. Lengthen up through the spine but do not grip the neck. Slide the shoulder blades down the spine.

2 Inhale and tilt your pelvis to create a C-shaped spine. Keeping your feet flat on the floor, roll down bone by bone, creating space between the vertebrae. Your hands are there to support you if you lose control but try to rely on abdominal strength to stabilize the movement.

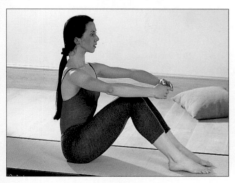

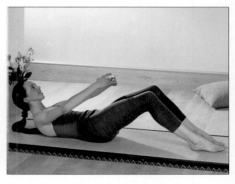

3 This time, hold your arms directly in front of you, level with your shoulders. Your elbows should be bent and arms rounded. Let your shoulder blades glide down your spine and feel the crown of your head 'float' up toward the ceiling. Inhale and tilt your pelvis to begin the downward roll as before.

4 When you first progress to this position try a few small roll-downs first to get the feel of the movement before going down any farther. Feel the support of your abdominals throughout the downward and upward roll. Make sure that you keep your feet flat on the floor all the time.

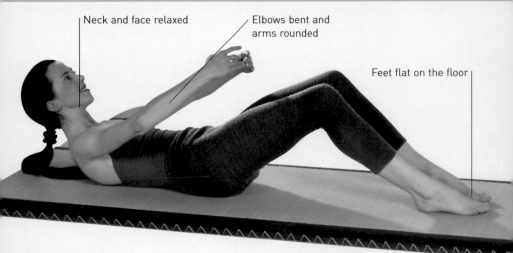

Neck and face relaxed

Elbows bent and arms rounded

Feet flat on the floor

Purpose
To strengthen the abdominals.

Target muscles
Abdominals, hip flexors.

Repetitions
Repeat 10 times.

Benefits
- This slow, controlled movement strengthens the abdominals.
- As your abdominals become stronger, you will be flatter and firmer and you will watch your wardrobe change.
- Regular roll-ups will allow your back to respond with comfort and ease.
- Your body will become gradually aligned, with optimum results.
- Eventually you will be free from the burden of aches and stiffness.
- Strengthening the abdominals will help you to improve your posture.
- Once the abdominals and back muscles are strong, they will support your torso without any effort.
- Your balance will improve and you will be able to do your exercises easily.

Checkpoints
- Do not overgrip the legs, use them only as support.
- Lengthen up through the spine in the starting position.
- Feel the abdominals pull you up.
- Use the abdominals, not momentum, to pull you up.
- Lower bone by bone.
- Keep the feet on the floor.
- Between each roll, lengthen up through the spine.
- As you curl down, imagine your spine is a bicycle chain that you are placing down link by link. When you have lowered down as far as you can, exhale and contract the abdominals to roll back up to the starting position. Sit upright, keeping your spine in neutral.
- Although you are curving your spine, do not collapse in to the movement.
- Roll down only a little way when you first try this exercise to get the feel of the movement, then roll lower as you become stronger.
- Do a mental check that you are not tensing your neck and face.

The Hundred

This exercise is one of the most commonly taught Pilates exercises. Challenge yourself to reach a hundred; the exercise really tests your co-ordination. Try to ensure that your breath is flowing and even.

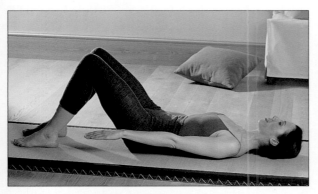

1 Lie on your back with bent knees, your feet flat and your head aligned. With a neutral spine and the abdominals hollowed, draw the navel to the spine. The arms are by your sides, lifted up. Slide the shoulder blades down your spine. Inhale to a count of five then exhale for five. Tap your fingers on the floor and co-ordinate breathing. with taps. Breathe steadily.

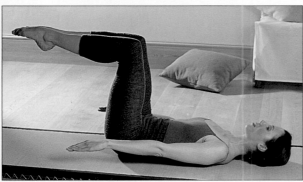

2 Next, lift the feet off the floor. Your knees should be directly above your hips and your feet level with your knees. Do not let your knees fall away or your spine will curve. If this is difficult, raise one leg, but do not twist the hips. Repeat the breathing pattern as before. Keep the abdominals flat and keep a distance between hips and ribs.

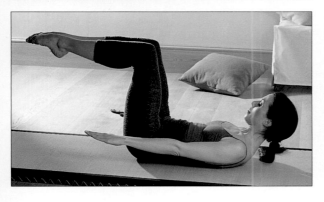

3 Curl the upper body off the floor. Drop the chin to your chest so that you are facing your thighs. Do not grip your neck and keep drawing the shoulder blades down your spine. Maintain the breathing pattern for a hundred beats. If you want a challenge, straighten your legs. Look to check that the abdominals are flat and your ribs are not flaring up.

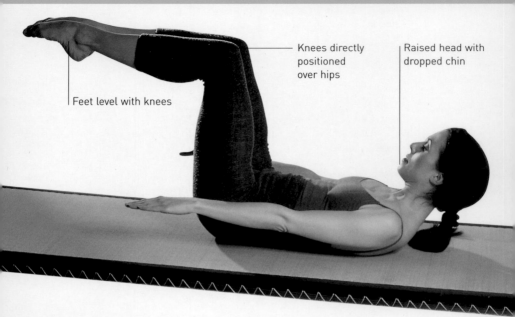

Raised head with dropped chin

Knees directly positioned over hips

Feet level with knees

Purpose

To strengthen core muscles, co-ordinate breathing patterns and build endurance. It can be used as a dynamic warm-up for the lungs and abdominals.

Target muscles

Transverse abdominis, rectus abdominis, stabilizing mid-back muscles.

Repetitions

20 x 5 beats.

Benefits

- This static contraction builds core strength by working on and strengthening the core muscles.
- By controlled breathing into your ribs, you can co-ordinate breathing patterns.
- The Hundred is a good test of general co-ordination.
- Regular exercising will build up endurance.

Checkpoints

- Keep your arms lengthened.
- Keep the abdominals hollowed.
- Don't grip your neck while you are drawing your shoulder blades down your spine.
- Keep your knees above your hips.
- Toes are pointed.
- Feet stay level with knees.
- Release tension from the neck.
- Do not clench your jaw.
- Keep the abdominals flat.
- Pay special attention to any tension in the neck and face in this position.
- To help you do this exercise well, visualize a heavy weight balancing on your abdominals so that your abdomen is flat and the weight is pulling your navel down toward your spine.
- Breathe steadily and imagine that you are breathing laterally into your ribs throughout the exercise.
- If you have neck or back problems, keep the knees bent and the feet flat on the floor throughout the exercise.

The Swimming

This exercise is a favourite with physiotherapists as it is a very effective way of developing strength in the core muscles. It is a challenging exercise but is an easy one to cheat on, so read the instructions carefully.

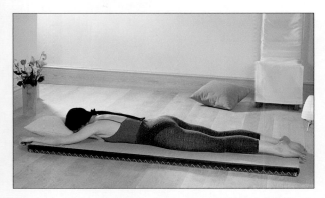

1 Lie on your front, placing a small pillow under your forehead to keep your head in alignment with your spine, which is in the neutral position. Keep the neck long. Stretch your arms over your head and lengthen them away. Point your toes and lengthen your legs away. Breathe laterally, wide and full. Draw in your abdominals.

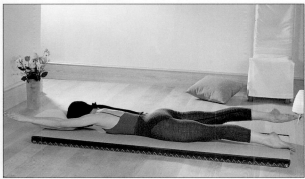

2 Introduce a challenge to your core strength by lifting one leg. Exhale as you lift and inhale as you lower the leg. Keep both hips in contact with the floor, and do not try to lift the leg too high. Keep lengthening as you lift, maintaining the distance between the ribs and hips. Do not lose the lift in your abdominals. Do not twist the raised leg.

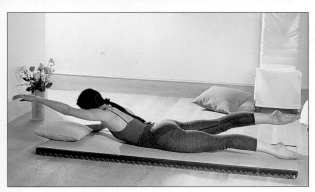

3 As you exhale, lift your opposite arm and leg together. When you lift your arm raise your head and upper body with the movement, but keep facing the floor so that your head stays in line with your spine. Lengthen through the arms and legs and keep your hips in contact with the floor. Imagine you have a drawing pin under the navel.

36

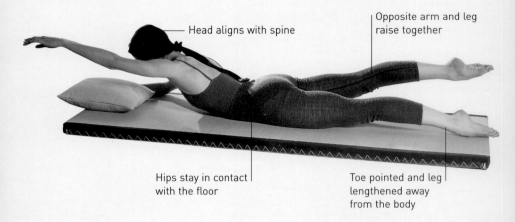

Head aligns with spine

Opposite arm and leg raise together

Hips stay in contact with the floor

Toe pointed and leg lengthened away from the body

Purpose
A strength exercise, challenging co-ordination and core strength.

Target muscles
Abdominals, gluteals, erector spinae.

Repetitions
Repeat 10 times.

Checkpoints
- Do not tip your head back.
- Keep the abdominals lifted.
- Breathe laterally.
- Lengthen as you lift the leg.
- Do not twist the hips.
- Keep your head in line with your spine.
- Do not twist the torso.
- Lengthen from a strong centre.
- Keep the head and the neck in line with the spine and working as extensions of the spine throughout.
- When you draw in the abdominals in the first position, imagine that there is a drawing pin on the mat that you are lifting away from.
- In position two, when you raise your leg, keep the knee and foot in line with your hips throughout.

Benefits
- An effective way of developing strength in the core muscles.
- The abdominals will become firmer, stronger and flatter.
- Like swimming, the exercise is a good workout for every part of the body. It is good for toning the abdominal muscles, the buttocks, back and hamstrings.
- The Swimming is a great counter exercise to front flexion exercises such as the Hundred.
- The exercise can be easily modified. You can divide the exercise between sessions so that you work with just the top or bottom half of your body.
- For anyone who has upper back and neck problems, only the lower half of the body need be worked. Keep your forehead on the mat and work the legs. Lengthen each leg, one at a time, so that they raise off the mat, then try the alternating leg movements.
- If you lose the lift in your abdominals, you will still benefit from the exercise if you continue to work in the second position for a while longer.

One Leg Stretch

Do not be fooled into thinking that this is a relaxing leg stretch – it is actually a very challenging movement which builds core strength and is also good for improving co-ordination. Keep your hips still throughout the exercise.

First position

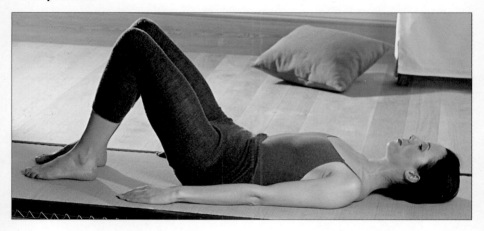

1 Lie on your back with your knees bent and your feet flat on the floor. Your spine should be in neutral and your head in alignment: do not shorten your neck by tipping your head back or dropping your chin to your chest. Draw the navel to the spine.

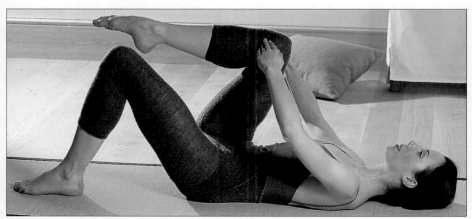

2 Lift one foot off the floor, keeping the knee bent, and pull the leg gently toward you, supporting it at the knee. Try not to overgrip, causing tension in the neck, and keep your foot in line with your knee. Take care not to let the ribs flare up. Repeat with the other leg.

Second position

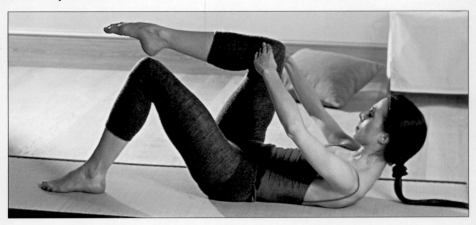

When the first position is understood, curl the upper body off the floor and continue the same movement. Let the chin fall toward the chest, and try to limit tension in the neck. Keep the hips very still, controlling any movement from the hips via your abdominals. Breathe laterally. Keep the stomach hollowed throughout the movement, trying to make it as flat as possible.

Third position

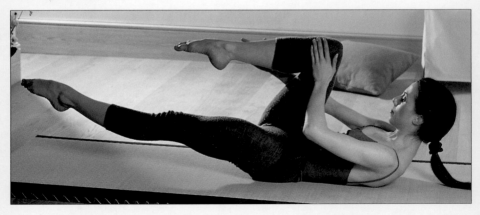

This position really challenges your co-ordination. As you raise the right leg, place the right hand on the ankle and the left hand on the inside of the knee. Change hands as you change legs. As one leg comes in to the body the other leg lifts and lengthens away on an exhalation. Keep your toes pointed and stretch down through the straight leg. The movement is controlled by the abdominals: keep them hollowed, and maintain the distance between the ribs and hips. Do not twist the hips: imagine they are being held in a vice. Keep the pace slow and consistent.

Leg Pull Prone

This is actually a yoga position as well as a modified Pilates position. You will gain a lot of torso strength and stability from this exercise, and if you do it properly it will feel as if every muscle in your body is being challenged.

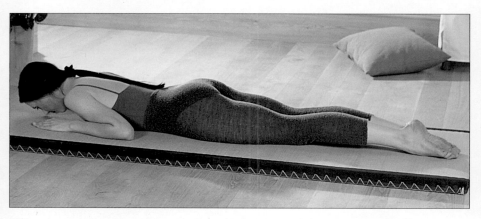

1 Lie on your front with your head in line with your spine. Bend your arms and keep your upper arms close to your body. Lift the abdominals off the floor, imagining that you are creating an arch under your stomach. Breathe wide and full. Concentrate on this abdominal lift and aim to hold it for 1 minute before relaxing again.

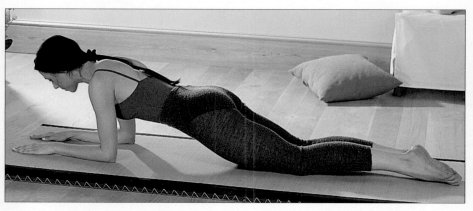

2 Your elbows should be directly under your shoulders. Do not push your buttocks toward the ceiling or arch your spine. Keep your head in line with the spine and lengthen it away; don't sink into your shoulders or squeeze the shoulder blades together. Make sure that your hips stay square. The abdominals are lifted throughout. If this is too difficult, lower your hips and curl just your upper body off the floor. Try to hold this position for at least 1 minute.

▶

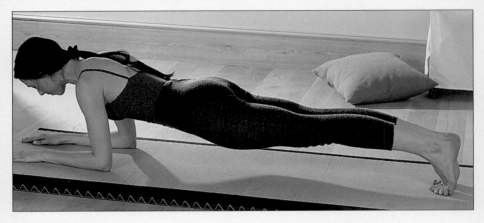

3 Lift up on to your toes, straightening your legs. This is a real challenge, so be sure to have worked on the first and second positions for quite some time before progressing. Take care not to transfer all the weight into your shoulders or upper body, and keep your hips square. Pull your navel to your spine, maintaining the distance between your ribs and hips, and breathe laterally. Aim to hold for up to 1 minute.

Purpose
To strengthen the abdominals and spine and challenge the upper body.

Target muscles
Abdominals, stabilizing back muscles.

Repetitions
Repeat up to 10 times.

Benefits
- Builds core strength
- A gain in torso strength and stability.
- Every muscle in the body will be engaged and challenged.
- Your back will feel more comfortable, with less aches and stiffness.
- The exercises help to align the body.
- Strengthening of the staples of Pilates – the abdominals and back.
- If you visualize a drawing pin inserted through your navel and attached to your back, you will focus on your abdominals, which stabilize the body.

Checkpoints
- Make sure your have mastered the first two positions before you attempt the third, which is quite a difficult movement to make.
- Slide your shoulders down your spine.
- Keep the upper arms close to your body.
- Maintain a straight line from your head to your knees.
- Do not let the abdominals sag.
- Do not transfer all your weight into your upper body.
- Draw your shoulder blades down your spine.
- Breathe freely throughout the exercise and do not hold your breath when holding the position.
- It is common to shrink down into your shoulders in this position so try to maintain the length in your neck throughout the movement.
- Keep checking for tension around the neck, face and shoulders.
- Focus on the abdominals throughout each position.

The Side-kick

This is another good exercise for core strength, concentrating on the lower body. Have patience and work gradually through the progressions to achieve the best results. Take care not to use momentum to lift and lower your leg.

First position

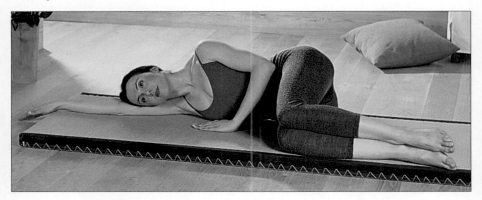

1 Lie on your side, resting your head on your outstretched lower arm. Keep your head in line with your spine, which is in neutral, and your hips stacked vertically: they must not roll in or out. Your knees are bent, one on top of the other. Place your free hand in front for balance but do not lean into the supporting arm or transfer your weight forward.

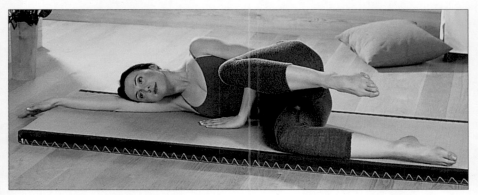

2 Lift the top knee directly above the other knee. Inhale and, with your toes pointed, move the knee back as you exhale until it travels behind your body. The challenge is to keep your hips stacked and at the same time ensure that your abdominals are hollowed. Your shoulder blades should be pulled down your spine and your ribs should not be pushed up. You should feel this in your side. If you want to increase the challenge, straighten the top leg, keeping the toe pointed.

42

Second position

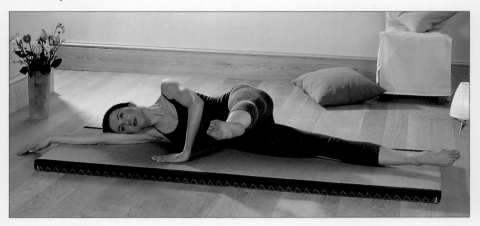

Straighten both legs. This is very challenging so be sure to advance only after working with the previous position first. Bring the bottom leg forward slightly from your hip, it should not be in line with your spine. Keep the hips vertical and lengthen out through both legs. The control comes from your centre. Exhale as the leg travels backward.

Purpose
To challenge core strength and work the lower body.

Target muscles
Hamstrings, hip flexors, abdominals, stabilizing shoulder muscles, abductors.

Repetitions
Repeat 10 times each side.

Benefits
- Strengthens and tones hips and legs.
- Develops core strength.
- Exercises help the body find its natural line and balance.
- Joints become stronger and more supple, while muscles get stronger and therefore more elastic.
- Balance is created between the muscles in the body, reducing tension.
- If your breathing is deep and steady, you will remove toxins from the body.

Checkpoints
- Do not transfer all your weight into the arm in front.
- Keep your abdominals flat.
- Do not let the hips collapse.
- Lengthen out through the legs.
- Visualize moving your leg through mud as this will slow you down and help to avoid using momentum to lift the leg.
- Your foot or knee should stay in line with your hip throughout.
- Move your legs slightly forward of the hips to maintain your balance and help to avoid injury to your lower back.
- Be aware of the alignment of your hips and keep them stacked on top of one another as it is common for the hips to roll forward and the posture to collapse. This movement is stabilized by your abdominals and the obliques (the muscles at the side of the waist). Try to keep a constant connection with their involvement.
- Control your breathing so that it is steady, and do not tense other parts of the body.

The Side-squeeze

This exercise will shape the waist and abdominals, so it is especially good for the area that hangs over your waistband. As you lift, check for tension in your neck or other parts of your body, and watch that your ribs stay down.

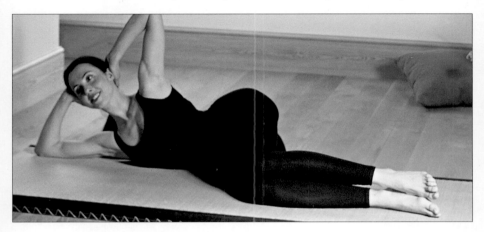

1 Lie on your side with your knees bent and in line with your hips. Your hips are stacked and your abdominals hollowed. Place your hands on your head, directly opposite each other. Do not tip your head back or drop your chin to your chest. Breathe in.

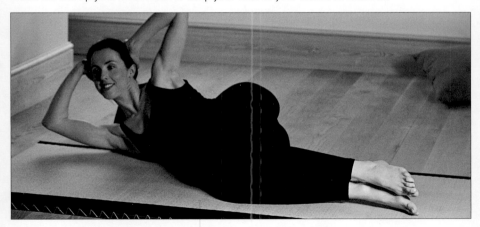

2 Exhale as you lift your upper body off the floor and inhale as you lower back down. Make the lift slow and controlled. Don't jerk your neck or grip too hard with your hands. Maintain the length through your spine and take care not to let your hips collapse, but keep them stacked. Make sure your knees stay level with your hips. Slowly draw your shoulder blades down your spine.

ABDOMINAL AND BACK EXERCISES

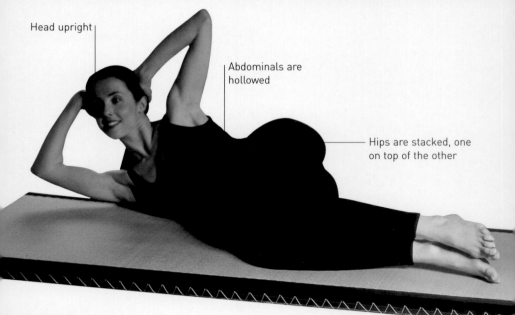

Head upright

Abdominals are
hollowed

Hips are stacked, one
on top of the other

Purpose
To strengthen the waist and mid-section,
stabilizing and improving balance.

Target muscles
Obliques, shoulder stabilizers, abdominals
and abductors.

Repetitions
Repeat 10 times on each side.

Benefits
- An increase in core strength, as well
  as becoming stronger all over.
- The abdominal muscles and waist
  will be shaped with this exercise.
- Your posture will improve.
- Some muscles are stretched, and
  some are lengthened.
- Once you exercise regularly, you
  will find that Pilates creates a lean,
  balanced body, thus reducing the
  risk of injury.

Checkpoints
- Do not allow the abdominals to sag; hold
  them taut throughout.
- Keep your hips stacked.
- Maintain the distance between your ribs
  and hips.
- Feel the muscles in your side working.
- Check for tension in the neck and other
  parts of the body, and relax if they feel
  under strain.
- Ensure that the ribs stay down.
- Check that you have good alignment and
  maintain it throughout the exercise; this
  is vital to make it effective.
- If you wish to add an extra challenge,
  raise the top knee, keeping it in line with
  your hips – no higher. Make this a slow,
  controlled movement.
- Take care not to overgrip with your
  hands. Perform the movement with flow,
  avoiding any jerky movements when
  lifting and lowering.

The Side Bend

This movement may look simple but it creates a marked improvement around the waistline if you practise it regularly, as well as developing core stability and balance. Feel the movement being controlled by your torso.

First position

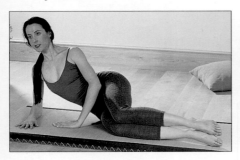 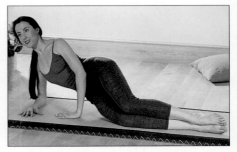

1 Lie on your side with the legs bent, knees level with hips and feet in line with the knees. Rest on your elbow, and bring the other arm in front for support.

2 Inhale, breathing laterally, and as you exhale lift your hips off the floor. Use the muscles in the side closest to the floor to control the movement via a strong centre.

Second position

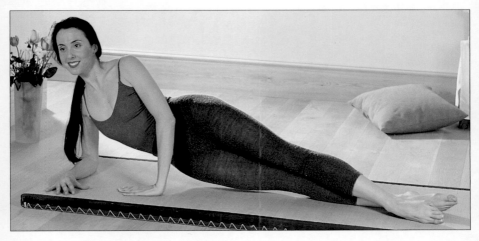

Progress only after reaching a level of ease in the first position. If you feel ready, straighten your legs and lengthen them away. Cross one foot over the other, with the toes pointed, to support you as you lift your hips. Keep your head in line with your spine and lengthen up through the top of your head.

46

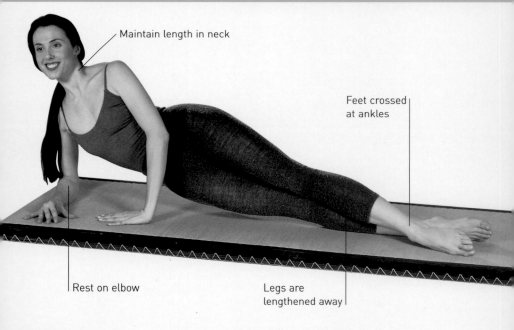

Maintain length in neck

Feet crossed at ankles

Rest on elbow

Legs are lengthened away

Purpose
To strengthen the abdominals and sides and improve balance.

Target muscles
Obliques, abdominals, stabilizing shoulder muscles and latissimus dorsi.

Repetitions
Repeat up to 10 times on each side.

Benefits
- A marked improvement in shape around the waistline.
- Develops core stability and balance.
- Improves lateral mobility of the spine.
- It targets the transversus abdominis and the oblique abdominal muscles.
- The exercise helps to loosen and stabilize the shoulder muscles and the upper chest muscles: the latissimus dorsi.

Checkpoints
- Initiate the movement via a strong centre.
- Control the movement using the torso.
- Do not transfer all your weight on to your arms.
- Keep the neck soft.
- Make sure the hips do not collapse either inward or outward. Imagine you have a red dot on your hips that always faces the ceiling as you lift.
- Keep the abdominals hollowed.
- Lift straight up, without veering to either side.
- Keep the movement flowing.
- To get real benefit, maintain correct alignment and try to perform the exercise accurately.
- Maintain the length in your neck and avoid sinking in to your shoulders.
- Be aware that you might find the exercise less challenging on one side than the other: one side may be stronger.
- Ensure that your ribs are not pushing up.

Push Ups

This is a classic exercise for shaping the upper body: the shoulders and biceps. If it is performed properly your abdominals will get a workout too. You can loosen up the spine by continuing the movement on the floor.

First position

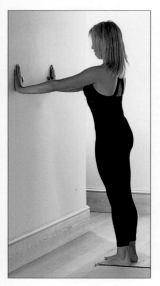

1 Stand facing a wall and place your hands on it. Your hands should be level with and just wider than your chest and flat against the wall, with the fingers pointing upward. Your feet stay flat on the floor. Keep the spine in neutral and lengthen up the body, feeling your head 'float' toward the ceiling.

2 Bend at the elbows to bring your chest toward the wall. Keep your head in line with your body, slide your shoulder blades down your spine, and ensure you are not pushing up your ribs.

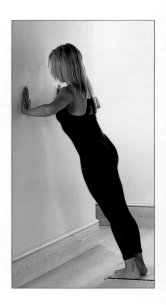

Second position

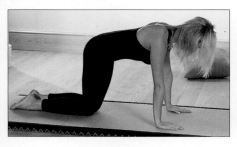

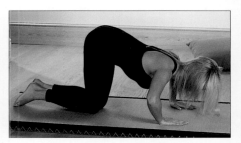

1 Position yourself on all fours, with your knees directly under your hips and hands directly under your shoulders, with the fingertips facing forward. Keep your spine in neutral and don't let your head sink into your neck.

2 Keeping your head in line with your spine, exhale as you lower your chest to the floor between your hands by bending your elbows. Do not allow the abdominals to sag. As you push up, straighten the arms without locking the elbows.

UPPER AND LOWER BODY EXERCISES

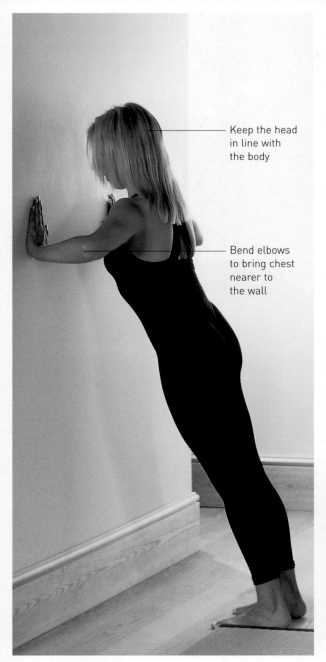

Keep the head in line with the body

Bend elbows to bring chest nearer to the wall

Purpose
To strengthen and shape the upper body.

Target muscles
Deltoids, pectorals, biceps, stabilizing back muscles and abdominals.

Repetitions
Repeat up to 10 times.

Checkpoints
- Keep your head in line.
- Do not let your head sink into your neck.
- Do not lock the elbows.
- Lower only as far as you can control.
- In the second position, keep your chest at hand level and your head forward of your hands. Ensure that you are not pushing up your ribs.
- In every position, pull the abdominals in, never allowing them to sag.
- Maintain your spine in neutral.
- Check for tension in your neck.
- Keep all your movement slow and controlled.

Benefits
- Push ups are perfect for shaping the upper body, the shoulders and biceps.
- Works out the abdominal muscles.
- The floor exercises mobilize the spine.
- Generally strengthens the upper body.

UPPER AND LOWER BODY EXERCISES

Third position

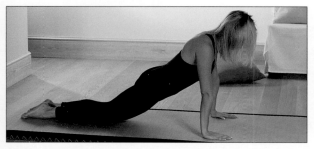

1 Drop your hips so that there is a straight line from your head to your knees. Your fingertips should be facing forward and your hands should be directly under the shoulders. Keep the abdominals strong and your hips square.

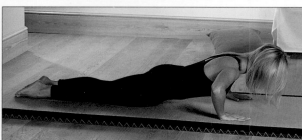

2 Exhale as you lower to the floor and inhale as you lift your body up. Keep your head in line with your spine and forward of your hands. Don't let your ribs flare up. Keep your weight evenly distributed between your knees and your hands.

Fourth position

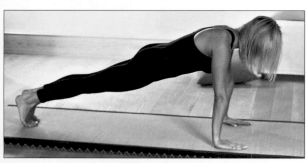

1 Form a straight line from your head to your feet, while supporting yourself on your toes and hands. The fingertips should face forward and your head should remain in alignment with your spine.

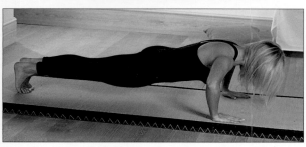

2 Lower your chest to the floor between your hands, then push up, keeping your elbows soft. Keep the movement controlled and continuous. Lower only as far as you can control.

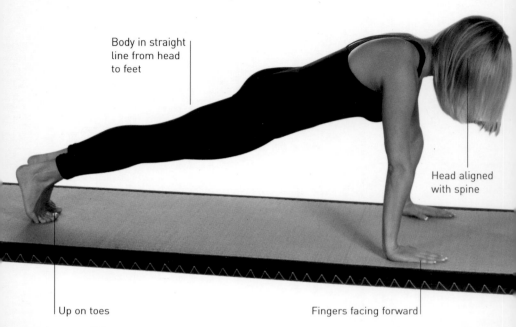

Body in straight line from head to feet

Head aligned with spine

Up on toes

Fingers facing forward

Checkpoints for third position
- Keep a straight line from your head to your knees.
- Do not let your buttocks stick up.
- Do not arch or curve your back.

Checkpoints for fourth position
- Keep your shoulder blades down the spine.
- Make it a controlled, flowing movement.
- Breathe laterally.
- Don't let your ribs flare up.
- Keep your abdominal muscles contracted throughout the exercise.
- Do not hold your breath at any time.
- Try to identify tension in muscles, especially in those that are not involved in the movement. Relax any muscles that are tense, for example the jaw and shoulders, which are commonly tensed.
- Listen to your body and stop if any area feels uncomfortable or causes pain.

- If you simply cannot focus on a position during a session, choose a similar exercise or one from the same category; don't waste your time and create negative feeling for a movement.

Benefits
- Engages core strength and helps to stabilize the whole torso and pelvis.
- Works the pectoral muscles and the arms.
- Gives the whole body a workout.
- The strength and control of stabilizing muscles are improved.
- The exercises help to realign and balance the body.
- Your body will become longer and leaner, and more toned.
- Your posture will improve, so you will appear to have lost weight.

Tricep Push Ups

A common complaint is the lack of muscle tone at the back of the upper arm: this exercise is excellent for challenging this area. It works by adapting the classic push-up to work on the triceps, but there are important differences.

First position

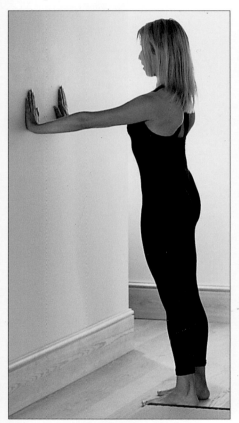 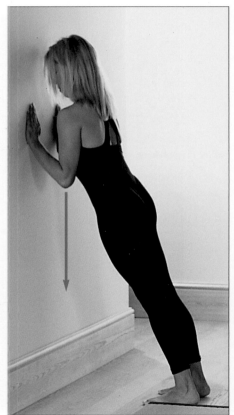

1 Stand facing a wall, positioning yourself an arm length away. Place your hands flat against the wall, with the fingers pointing upward. Your hands should be level with and just a little wider than your chest width. Your feet stay flat on the floor. Keep your spine in neutral and slide your shoulder blades down.

2 Bend at the elbows to bring your chest toward the wall as you exhale. Unlike the classic push up, your elbows should remain close to the body and pointing down at all times. Keep your head in line with your body and check that you are not pushing up your ribs. Push away from the wall to come back to your starting position.

Second position

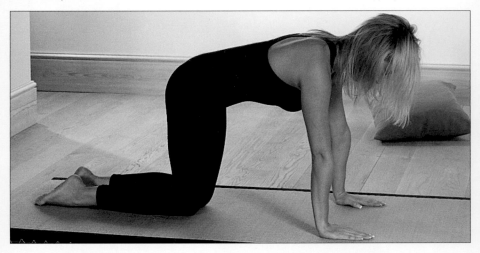

1 Position yourself on all fours, with your hands directly under your shoulders, fingertips facing forward. Keep your spine in neutral and maintain a straight line from your head to your hips. Don't let the abdomen sag.

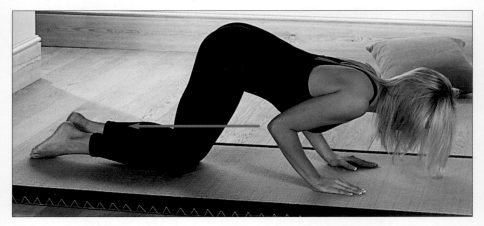

2 Exhale as you lower your chest to the floor. This time, bend at the elbow and ensure that your elbows do not point outward, but rather point toward your feet, with your upper arms staying as close to your sides as you can manage. As you push up, straighten the arms without locking the elbows.

Benefits
- Strengthens the upper body and the abdominals.
- Targets the triceps, pectorals, deltoids and abdominals.
- Defines muscles in upper arm.

Third position

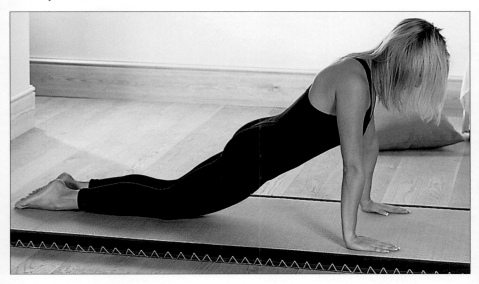

1 Drop your hips so that there is a straight line from your knees to your head. Glide your shoulder blades down your spine. Your fingertips should face forward.

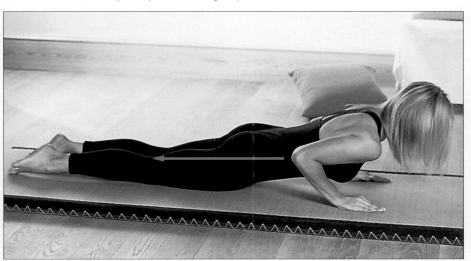

2 Exhale as you lower and inhale as you lift. Keep your head in line with your spine. Ensure that your head stays the same distance from your hands and that the elbows stay close to the body and pointing in the direction of your feet. Try to perform the exercise with flowing, continuous movements.

UPPER AND LOWER BODY EXERCISES

Fourth position

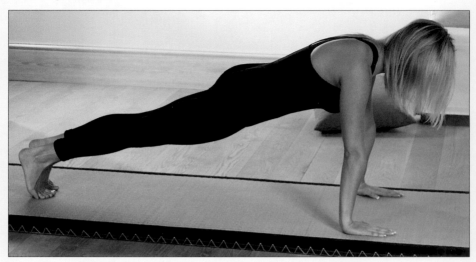

Make sure you have been practising the modified positions for some time before you progress to this position. This time your whole body should be in one straight line. Don't let your head sink in to your shoulders. Lower the chest to the floor, keeping your elbows pointing toward your feet and using the same breathing pattern as for the previous positions. Repeat up to 10 times.

Checkpoints for first position
- Do not let your elbows 'wing' out to the sides; they should stay close to the body. To help you keep your elbows in to your sides, visualize doing the movement in a narrow space between two walls. Maintain a constant, and slow, speed throughout the exercise, although this can be difficult to maintain on the last few repetitions.
- Watch for your shoulders moving up toward your ears.
- Lengthen up through the top of your head.

Checkpoints for second position
- Keep your chest level with your hands.
- The head should be forward of the hands.
- Ensure that your feet are flat on the floor.

Checkpoints for third position
- Do not let your buttocks stick up.
- During the push up, feel the movement

in the muscles in the back of your upper arms.
- Do not rely on momentum.

Checkpoints for fourth position
- You should really feel this in the triceps.
- Keep your body in alignment.
- Hollow the abdominals.
- Maintain a straight line from your head to your feet.

Benefits
- These exercises help to improve the muscle tone at the back of the upper arm: these positions challenge this area.
- The classic push up is adapted to specifically work on the triceps muscles at the top of the arms.

Tricep Dips

This exercise is good for firming up the muscles at the back of the arms. The tricep runs from the shoulder to the elbow and can be hard to work, but if neglected, this is the part of your arm that wobbles when you wave.

First position

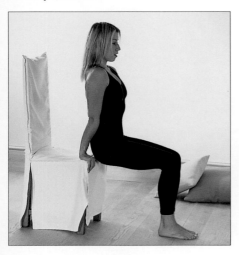

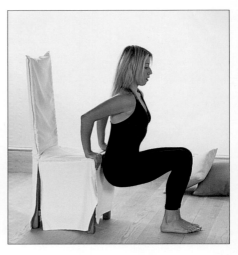

1 Place yourself in front of a chair with bent knees and feet flat on the floor. Support yourself on your hands with your fingers pointing forward.

2 Bend your elbows and lower your body as you inhale. Glide your shoulder blades gently down your spine and watch that your ribs do not push up.

Second position

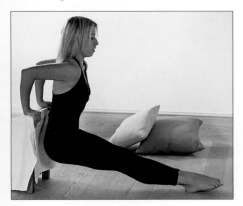

Start in the same basic position as above, but this time put your legs straight out in front of you with your toes pointed. Keep your back close to the chair, your elbows pointing straight behind you and fingers downward. In this advanced position it is very tempting to let the elbows travel out to the sides, particularly if you are tired, or not paying full attention. Ensure that your head does not sink in to your shoulders and remember to breathe fully. Your breathing should be wide and full, allowing your ribs to expand fully, but keep your abdominals hollowed out throughout the exercise.

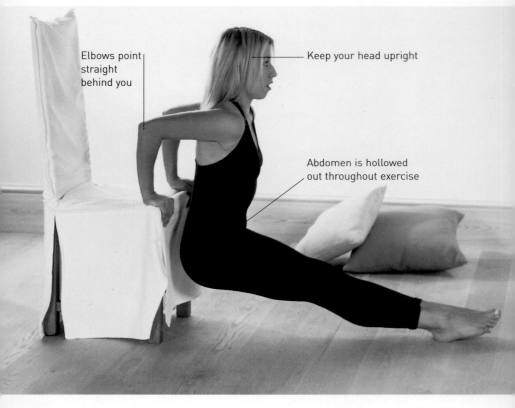

Elbows point straight behind you

Keep your head upright

Abdomen is hollowed out throughout exercise

Purpose
To tone the triceps.

Target muscles
Triceps, abdominals.

Repetitions
Start gently but work up to 20 times.

Benefits
- If you do this exercise regularly, you will see the back of the arms firming up. The flesh that wobbles will become more toned.
- Because the abdominals are kept hollowed, they will also benefit.

Checkpoints
- Lengthen up through your spine, which is in neutral. This is your starting position.
- Keep your back close to the chair.
- Do not lock your elbows, just straighten them.
- Ensure that elbows travel backward rather than out to the sides.
- Keep your head in line and ensure that it does not sink in to the shoulders.
- Do not use momentum.
- Keep the abdominals hollowed throughout the whole exercise.
- Maintain an even flow and aim to keep the movement continuous.
- Don't allow your pace to speed up or down; in this way you will work the muscle harder and get the maximum benefit.

The Outer Thigh Blaster

If practised regularly, this exercise will really firm up the outsides of the hips and thighs and strengthen the lower body. Do not let the abdominals sag, and slide your shoulder blades gently down your spine.

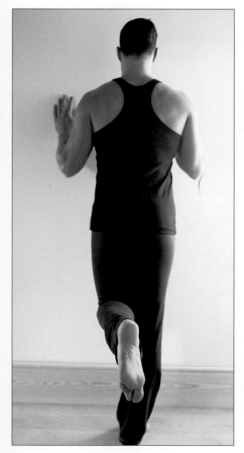 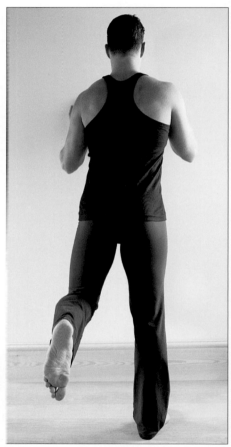

1 Stand facing the wall with the hands at chest level and flat against the wall. Bend one leg at the knee so that your foot is level with your knee and both knees are in line. Your spine should be in neutral and your foot flexed. Check that there is a straight line from your head to your feet and try not to lean in to the wall or bend at the hip.

2 From this starting position, take your knee out to the side. It is important to keep your foot flexed and your knees aligned. Exhale as your leg travels away from your body, then inhale as you bring it back. You should not swing the leg. Don't 'sink' in to the supporting leg, but keep lengthening up through the spine.

The Inner Thigh Lift

This is a popular exercise that is often done badly. However, when it is performed correctly it works wonders with that much complained about area, the inner thigh. To progress the exercise you could use ankle weights.

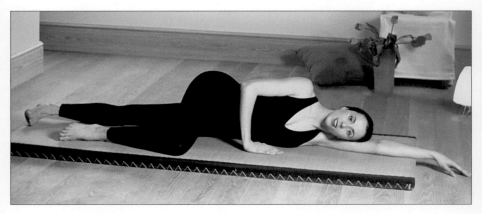

1 Lie on your side, supporting your head on your outstretched arm. Your hips should be stacked and your other hand can rest in front of you on the floor for support. Bend the top leg and rest your knee on the floor. Straighten the lower leg and lengthen it away on the floor with the foot flexed. Do not curve your back or allow your ribs to jut forward. Glide your shoulder blades down your spine.

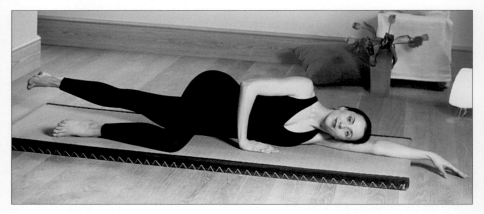

2 Inhale and, as you exhale, lift the bottom leg as high as you can, keeping the abdominals hollowed all the time, then lower it. Make the movement flow, trying to avoid any jerky movements or, worst of all, swinging your leg. You should feel the muscle of the inner thigh doing the work. Take care not to twist the knee. Keep your foot in line with your leg: there is a tendency to lead with the toes in this position.

The Open V

This is not one of the most graceful-looking movements, but it works wonders for the thighs, especially the inner thighs, and also benefits the abdominals. Keep your knees above your hips at all times.

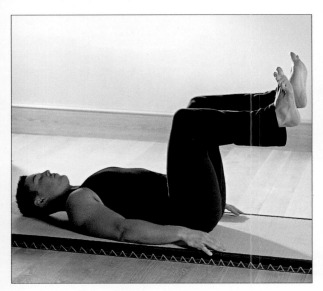

1 Lie on your back, with your knees bent and directly above your hips, and your feet level with your knees. Your feet should be flexed. The arms are on the floor, lengthening away, your shoulder blades slide down your spine, and your head is in alignment with your spine. Start with your knees apart and keep them directly above your hips. Don't let them drop to the floor or your lower back may curve upward and could cause stress. Try not to hold any tension in your neck and shoulders, but stay as relaxed as you can.

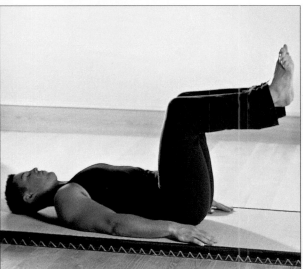

2 Keeping your feet in line with your knees, bring your knees together and squeeze to feel your inner thighs working. Hold for a few seconds, then return to the starting position. Keep your abdominals hollowed throughout and your spine in neutral.

Benefits
- The inner thighs will become toned and firm.
- The hip, back and abdominal muscles will be exercised.

UPPER AND LOWER BODY EXERCISES

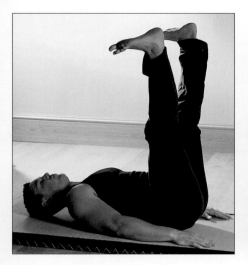

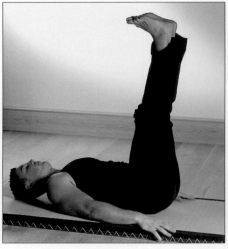

1 The basic movement is the same as before in the first position, but it is done with straight legs. Lengthen up through your heels and keep your feet flexed. Start with your legs apart.

2 Bring your legs together and squeeze to work your inner thighs. Keep the hips still via the abdominals, which are hollowed throughout. Keep your arms strong, and really feel your inner thighs working.

Benefits
- Targets adductors, hip flexors, abdominals and stabilizing back muscles.
- Firms up inner thighs.

Checkpoints
- Do not allow your legs to drop away from your body.
- Do not let the legs open too far.
- Squeeze the knees together.
- Watch for tension in the neck.
- Lengthen the arms away.
- Lengthen up through the heels.
- Slide your shoulder blades down your spine.
- Watch that your ribs do not flare up.
- Keep hollowing the abdominals: you can glance down and check that they are held flat. Squeeze the legs together as before.

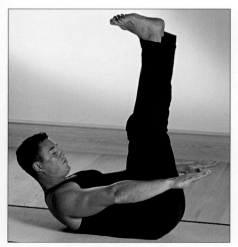

3 Curl the upper body off the floor, watching for tension in the neck and shoulders. Don't let your head sink in to your shoulders, but glide your shoulder blades down your spine.

Feet and Ankle Exercises

This movement will improve your balance and strengthen your lower body
and all the small muscles in your feet and ankles – it is great for weak
ankles. Initially, you may find the balance quite challenging.

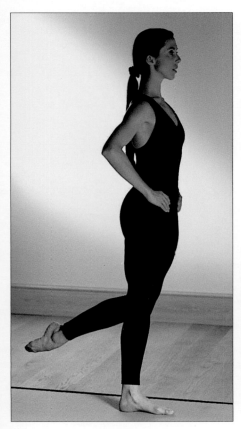
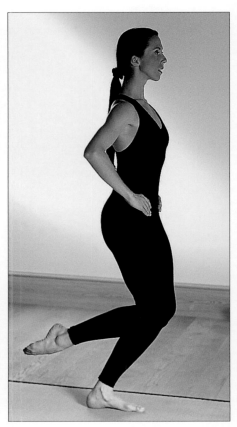

1 Stand up tall and imagine the crown of your head floating up to the ceiling. Feel your spine lengthening. It should stay in neutral throughout. Keep your abdominals as flat as possible. Place your hands on your hips and keep the head in line with your spine. Keeping your knees in line with one another, let one foot hover above the floor as you balance evenly on the other.

2 Bend the supporting leg and lower your body as far as you can control. Do not collapse in to the movement. The supporting foot may feel a little wobbly at first. Check that the knee of the supporting leg stays in alignment with the foot. Inhale as you come back up to standing. Keep your upper body strong and watch that your ribs do not travel away from your hips.

▶

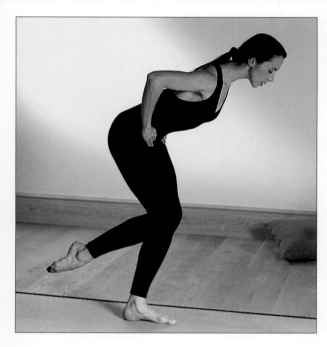

3 Bend your knee and lower as far as you can in to the position as before. This time, you are going to hold this position and then very carefully lower your chest toward the floor. Bend only a little initially. To get back to the starting position, straighten your torso first then come back up to standing. Keep your head in line with your spine.

Purpose
To strengthen lower body, feet and ankles.

Target muscles
Quadriceps, supporting muscles around feet and ankles, abdominals.

Repetitions
Repeat up to 10 times on each leg.

Benefits
- Affects both the upper and lower body.
- All the small muscles in the feet and ankles will be strengthened. It is especially good for weak ankles.
- The lower body will gain strength.
- With practice, balance will be much improved.
- Any subtle differences in strength will be balanced out.

Checkpoints
- Watch for your knees rolling inward or outward and correct it as soon as you notice a problem.
- Keep your supporting foot flat on the floor throughout the exercise.
- Lengthen up through the spine.
- Try to make the movement smooth and continuous.
- Do not try to lower too far.
- Do not collapse into the movement.
- Keep lifting the abdominals.
- If you find it difficult to balance, it may help to look at a fixed point on the wall. It is common to find that your balance is better on one side than the other because most people favour one side over the other.
- Concentrate on maintaining the alignment between your foot and knees during all the exercises here. It may help to visualize your supporting leg being held between two narrow walls.

63

One Leg Kick

This core exercise really challenges your co-ordination as you cannot see the movement – you just feel it. It is fantastic for toning up the lower body while at the same time challenging core strength.

First position

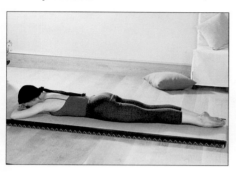

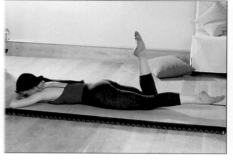

1 Lie on your front, supporting your forehead on your folded hands to keep the head in alignment. Draw your navel to your spine, trying to form an arch under your abdominals.

2 Relax the neck and avoid clenching the jaw. Relax your shoulders and slide the shoulder blades down your spine. Bend one leg at the knee. This is your starting position.

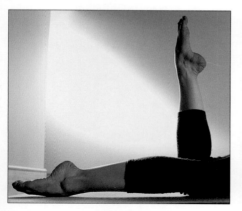

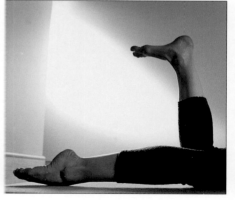

3 Inhale slowly, and, as you start to exhale, point your toes and make a stabbing movement with your foot toward your buttocks, so that the foot faces the ceiling. Keep your knees together and lengthen through the legs.

4 Ease out of this position then repeat, this time with your foot in a flexed position. Then extend your leg back to its original position. Meanwhile, the supporting leg on the floor should be lengthening away at all times.

Second position

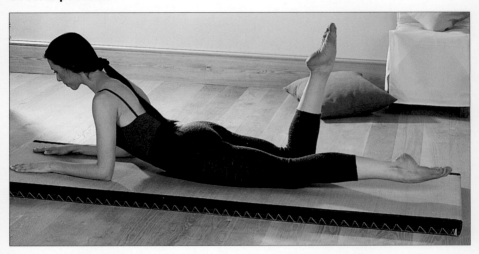

Perform the same movements, but this time curl your upper body off the floor and rest on your elbows. Slide the shoulder blades down. Keep your neck long throughout and watch that your ribs do not travel away from your hips. Lengthen through the spine. If you feel a pinch in your spine in this position, stay with the first position for a while.

Purpose
To tone the lower body and to help to develop core stability and strength.

Target muscles
Hamstrings, erector spinae (when upper body is lifted), abdominals and gluteals.

Repetitions
Repeat 10 times with each leg.

Benefits
- Tones the lower body and helps to develop core strength.
- Works and strengthens the hamstrings and glutes; resist just placing the leg; force the hamstrings to do it.
- Strengthens upper arms and also stretches quadriceps and the abdominal muscles.

Checkpoints for first position
- Keep the movement swift and continuous.
- Limit any movement by keeping the abdominals hollowed throughout.
- Slide the shoulder blades down your spine.
- If your quadricep muscles are tight, don't bend your knee farther than is comfortable or repeat too many times.

Checkpoints for second position
- Keep your neck in line throughout the exercise.
- Breathe wide and full.
- Do not push all your weight into your arms.
- A good way to visualize the movement is to imagine that you are squeezing a pillow between your hamstrings and your calf.
- You may find it easier to get a feel for the movement first, then add the correct breathing pattern and work on lengthening down through the other leg.

Spine Stretch

If your back feels tight or if you just want to achieve a healthy and mobile spine then this is the stretch for you. You will feel longer, stretched and more flexible. This is a flowing movement rather than a static stretch.

First position

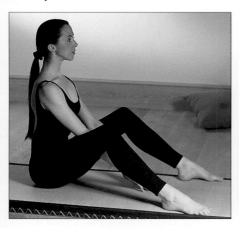
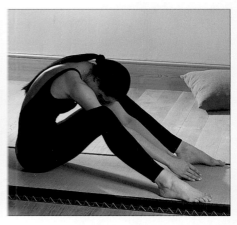

1 Sit upright with your knees bent and your feet flat on the floor. Create as much length through your spine as possible so that you can make your stretch as effective as possible. Try not to tense your neck and keep the shoulders relaxed.

2 Let your chin drop to your chest, then roll down bone by bone through your spine. As you do so, gently reach forward with your hands. Keep your abdominals hollowed throughout. Roll back up to the starting position and lengthen through the spine.

Second position

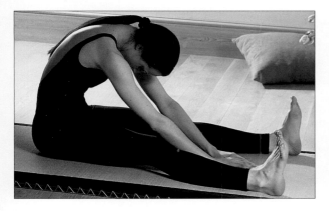

The movement is the same as before, but this time straighten the legs and flex your feet, lengthening the heels away. Bend the knees slightly if you find this uncomfortable. The legs should be parted as far as is comfortable. As you roll up, try to create as much length as possible between the vertebrae. Keep your buttocks on the floor during the exercise.

STRETCHES

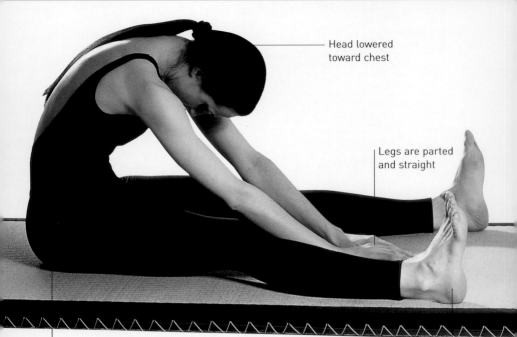

Head lowered
toward chest

Legs are parted
and straight

Buttocks on the floor

The feet are flexed

Purpose
To stretch the spine.

Target muscles
Erector spinae, hamstrings, adductors
and abdominals.

Repetitions
Repeat 10 times.

Benefits
- Helps to loosen up your back if it
  feels tight.
- Stretches out your spine, making it
  feel longer, stretched and more flexible.
- Works the abdominal muscles and
  upper leg muscles.

Checkpoints
- Do not collapse into the stretch; lift up
  through the abdominals and spine. Exhale
  as you lower in to the stretch.
- Keep the movement flowing and
  continuous; this is not a static stretch.
- Let your head float up to the ceiling.
- Do not have the legs too far apart.
- Roll up vertebra by vertebra.
- Imagine that you have a large beach ball
  in front of you, and lift up and over the
  ball. As you come upright again, imagine
  that your back is rolling up a pole,
  vertebra by vertebra, and take care to
  keep this alignment from your head
  to your hips: do not lean forward or away
  from the imaginary pole.
- If stretching out the legs is too much of a
  strain, bend the knees slightly.

Spine Twist

A deceptively challenging movement, this twist will stretch the waist and lower back while strengthening the abdominals. To gain the maximum benefit, keep your bottom on the floor throughout this movement.

First position

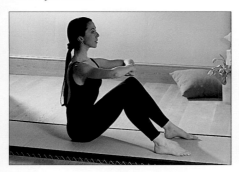

1 Sit upright, lengthening up through the spine, with your knees bent and feet flat on the floor, legs slightly apart. Cross your arms loosely across your chest. Maintain a straight line from your head to your bottom.

2 Breathing laterally, inhale and, as you exhale, turn the upper body to one side, keeping your buttocks on the floor. Repeat on the other side. Remember that this is a flowing movement, not a static position.

Second position

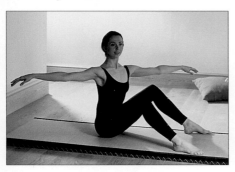

The basic movement is the same but with straight arms, lengthening out through the arms from the shoulders. Take care not to drop them. Now you are stretching in two directions: lengthening out through your arms and up through your spine. Slide the shoulder blades gently down your back.

Third position

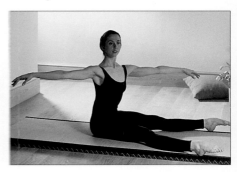

The movement is the same but this time straighten the legs and point your toes. You are now stretching in three directions: up through your spine, out through your arms and through your legs. Be sure to keep your buttocks on the floor. You may be tempted to lean in to one side as you turn.

68

STRETCHES

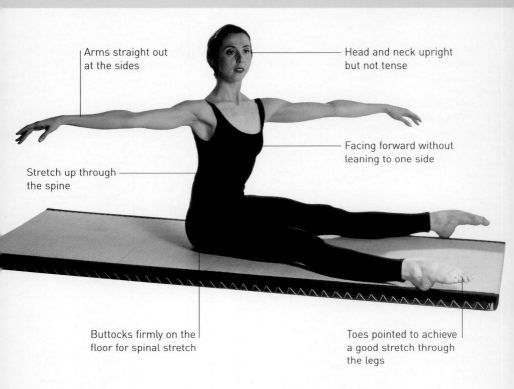

Arms straight out at the sides

Head and neck upright but not tense

Facing forward without leaning to one side

Stretch up through the spine

Buttocks firmly on the floor for spinal stretch

Toes pointed to achieve a good stretch through the legs

Purpose
To stretch the sides, strengthen the abdominals and promote thoracic mobility.

Target muscles
Obliques, abdominals, adductors and hamstrings.

Repetitions
Repeat 10 times on each side.

Benefits
- Stretches the waist and lower back.
- Strengthens the abdominals.
- Mobilizes the chest area.
- Works several muscles at the same time; in the abdomen, upper legs and at the sides of the abdomen.

Checkpoints
- Keep the movement flowing.
- Hollow the abdominals.
- Lengthen up through the spine.
- Do not collapse into the movement.
- Keep the whole of your buttocks on the floor.
- Do not curve the spine.
- Lengthen all the way to the toes.
- Feel the abdominals working.
- Try to keep the movement smooth and continuous.
- Try to consciously sit correctly aligned. Certain postural habits can develop, which are challenged by this particular exercise so it may feel very intense at first. It does get easier wth practice.
- It is important to position your feet correctly; either flat on the floor or with the toes pointed.

Lower Back Stretch

This is a good warm-up stretch. Taking deep breaths can help you to relax
in to the stretch and you may find your muscles becoming more pliable,
allowing you to ease yourself further into the movement.

First position

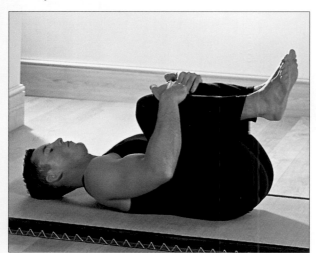

Lie on your back and bring both knees up toward your chest. Support your legs with your hands, just below your knees. Relax your shoulders and feel the stretch in your lower back. Remember to keep your abdominals hollowed. Inhale to prepare and exhale as you lift your legs.

Second position

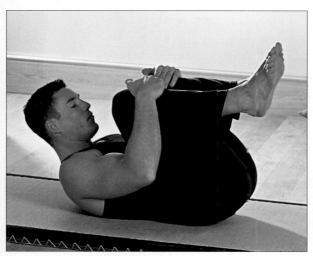

Curl your head and shoulders off the floor, imagining curling up like a ball. Keep your neck soft: do not force your head forward to your knees. Take care not to overgrip – keep your elbows open.

Focus

Some people find it beneficial to rock from side to side in this stretch to gently mobilize the lower back.

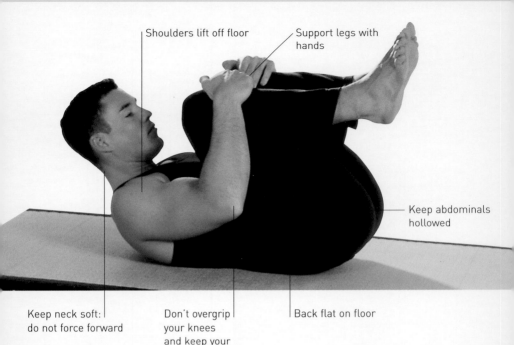

Shoulders lift off floor

Support legs with hands

Keep abdominals hollowed

Keep neck soft: do not force forward

Don't overgrip your knees and keep your elbows open

Back flat on floor

Purpose
To stretch the lower back.

Target muscles
Erector spinae and gluteals.

Repetitions
Stretch twice; hold for 30 seconds each.

Benefits
- This exercise is good when used as a warm-up stretch.
- Can ease mild tension in the lower back.
- Gently mobilizes the lower back.
- This stretch can be done anywhere if you have a mat or a rug to lie on.
- Works the erector spinae and gluteal muscles in the lower back.

Checkpoints
- Check for tension in the neck and shoulders and try not to hold them rigidly.
- Relax in to the stretch.
- Do not overgrip with your hands.
- Curl up and down slowly.
- Make sure your mat is thick enough to protect your back.
- If you are quite stiff, you can gently mobilize the lower back by rocking slightly from side to side while you are doing this stretch. To do this, keep your upper body on the floor and make the movement very subtle.
- Although a number of repetitions are recommended, these are only a guideline until you are confident about your mobility.
- Hold the stretch for longer or repeat if you need to.

Spine Press

This movement mobilizes and stretches the lower spine. It is a good one to try whenever your lower back feels stiff, especially if you have been sitting for a long period, at your desk for example – and it can be done very discreetly.

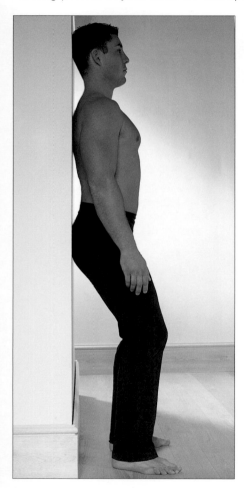 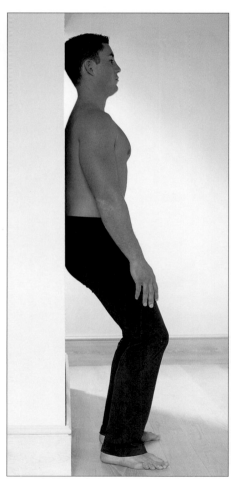

1 Stand a short distance away from a wall, with your back against the wall, your knees bent and your arms by your sides. Lengthen up and glide your shoulder blades down your spine. If you have problems with your lower back, do step 2 only.

2 Inhale and, as you exhale, push your spine flat against the wall by tilting your pelvis and contracting your abdominals. Keep your head in alignment. Try not to collapse into the movement: keep your abdominals hollowed and the spine lengthened.

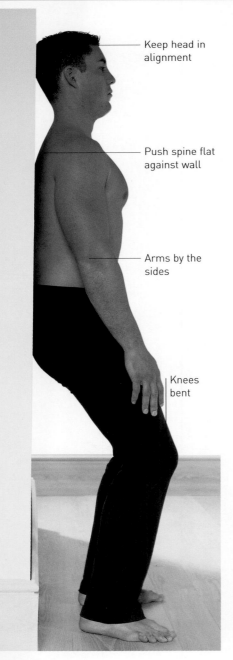

Keep head in alignment

Push spine flat against wall

Arms by the sides

Knees bent

Purpose
To mobilize and stretch the muscles in lower back.

Target muscles
Erector spinae and abdominals.

Repetitions
Stretch twice; hold each movement for about 30 seconds.

Checkpoints
- Do not curve your spine too much, the curvature should be very subtle.
- Too much curving of the spine can 'pinch' the muscles in the lower back.
- If curving your spine is uncomfortable, or if you have ongoing problems in your lower back, just perform the second part of the movement only. If you experience any pain during the exercise, don't carry on, and wait a while before trying it again.
- Avoid collapsing in to the movement by lengthening your spine; use slow, measured movements to avoid overstraining your muscles.
- Keep the abdominals hollowed throughout the movement; they need to be strong to support the spine.
- When you tilt your pelvis, initiate the movement by visualizing that you are pressing your navel in the direction of your spine.
- Keep your head in alignment during the movement.

Benefits
- Stretches and mobilizes the lower back.
- Targets and works the abdominal muscles and muscles in the lower back.
- The exercise can easily and quickly be done at home or in the office to counteract sitting for long periods at a desk.

Chest Stretch

This feel-good stretch uses a wall for support. It is great for relieving tightness in the chest and it can be done almost anywhere to stretch the chest muscles and work the pectorals.

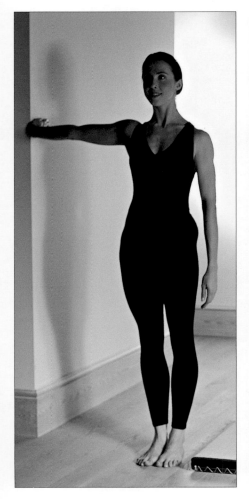 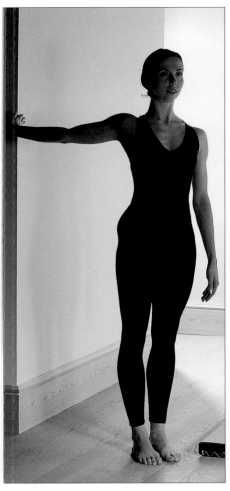

1 Stand sideways to a wall. Extend one arm and place your hand flat on it. Keep your hand in line with your chest and your feet in line with your hips. Draw in your abdominals; your spine stays in neutral.

2 Now turn your hips away from the wall, so that you can feel a stretch in your chest. Relax your shoulders and enjoy the stretch opening up the chest. Change sides and repeat the movement.

74

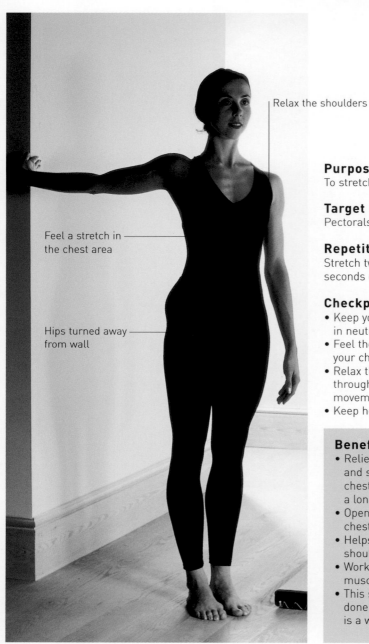

Relax the shoulders

Feel a stretch in the chest area

Hips turned away from wall

Purpose
To stretch the chest.

Target muscles
Pectorals.

Repetitions
Stretch twice; hold for 30 seconds each.

Checkpoints
- Keep your spine in neutral.
- Feel the stretch in your chest.
- Relax the shoulders throughout the movement.
- Keep head upright.

Benefits
- Relieves tightness and stiffness in the chest after sitting for a long time.
- Opens up the chest area.
- Helps to relax the shoulders.
- Works the pectoral muscles.
- This stretch can be done wherever there is a wall to rest on.

Gluteals Stretch

This stretch is reasonably easy to do and promotes a greater range of movement in the lower body. It is also a valuable stretch to do before many different sports that involve a lot of lower body work.

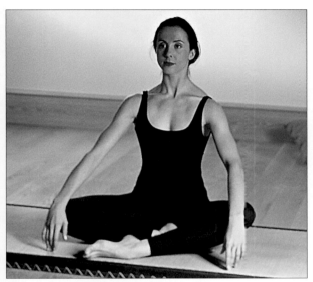

1 Sit on the floor and position one leg in front of the other (the legs are not crossed). Relax your arms in front of you. Lengthen up through the spine, creating space between the vertebrae. Don't worry if your knees don't fall to the floor, just relax and let the knees fall into a natural position.

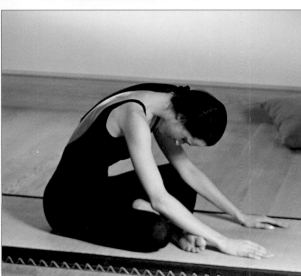

2 Drop your chin toward your chest and curl down the spine while pushing the arms forward and keeping your buttocks on the floor. Curl up again, switch the positions of the legs and repeat on the other side. Do not collapse into the movement; keep the abdominals pulled in throughout the exercise.

Focus
Make all your movements quite deliberate: don't be guided by momentum.

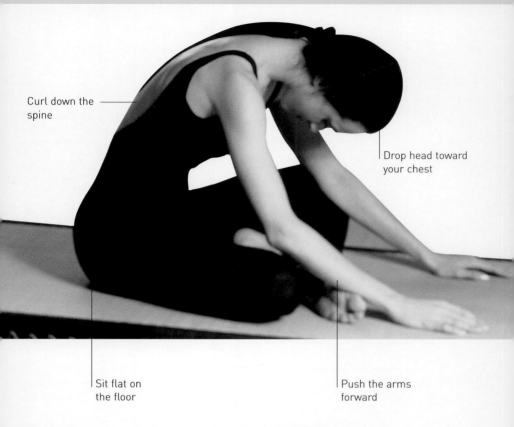

Curl down the spine

Drop head toward your chest

Sit flat on the floor

Push the arms forward

Purpose
To stretch the lower body.

Target muscles
Gluteals.

Repetitions
Stretch twice; hold for 30 seconds each.

Benefits
- Stretches the lower body.
- Targets the gluteal muscles.
- Promotes a greater range of movement in the lower body.
- Good stretch before sport.

Checkpoints
- Don't cross your legs, keep them slightly separate.
- Relax the arms in both positions.
- Try to create length between the vertebrae by lengthening up through the spine.
- Don't force your knees to fall to the floor; just relax and let them fall into a natural position.
- When performing the gluteals stretch, be sure to keep your buttocks on the floor or you will not stretch enough.
- Replace the spine bone by bone.
- Perform the stretch slowly and deliberately in a controlled way, rather than collapsing into it.

Deep Chest and Back Stretch

This stretch is ideal for easing tightness in the chest and back. Try to relax your shoulders and neck into the stretch. Remember, if this stretch is too intense, you can bend your knees.

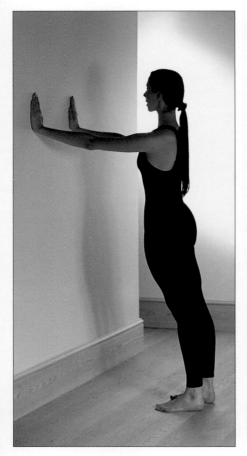

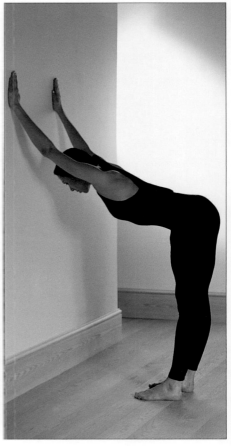

1 Stand facing the wall with your feet together and place your hands flat on the wall level with your shoulders, just wider than shoulder-width apart. Lengthen up through the spine.

2 Inhale, then as you exhale lower your chest by bending from the hips, to feel a stretch in your chest and back. Keep your head in line with your spine. Keep the spine lengthened and the abdominals hollowed.

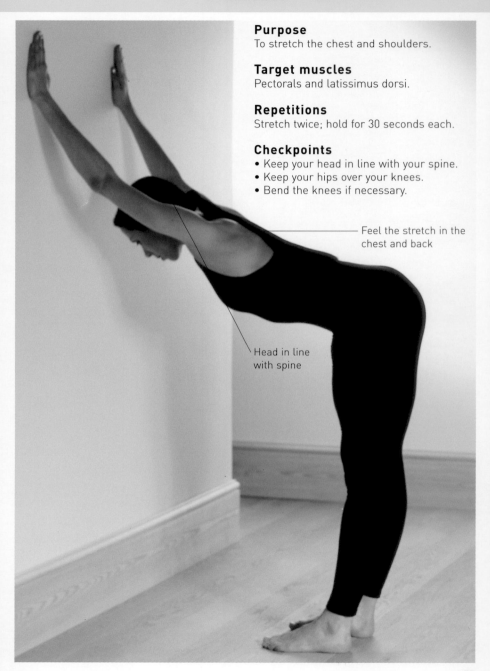

Purpose
To stretch the chest and shoulders.

Target muscles
Pectorals and latissimus dorsi.

Repetitions
Stretch twice; hold for 30 seconds each.

Checkpoints
• Keep your head in line with your spine.
• Keep your hips over your knees.
• Bend the knees if necessary.

Feel the stretch in the chest and back

Head in line with spine

Abdominal Stretch

This is a very popular stretch that is similar to the 'cobra' in yoga. It is good for stretching the abdominals. Take care not to throw your head back in this stretch. Keep facing the floor and lengthen up through the top of your head.

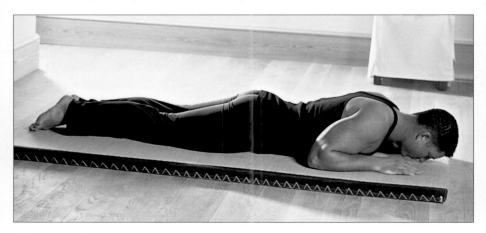

1 Drop your hips so that there is a straight line from your knees to your head. Glide your shoulder blades down your spine. Your fingertips should face forward.

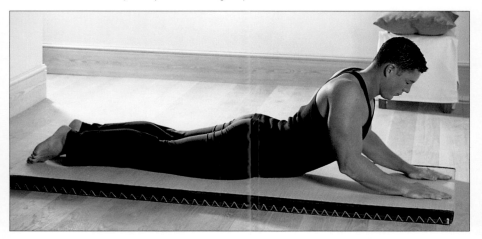

2 Inhale and, as you exhale, lift your upper body off the floor, resting the weight on your arms. Keep the abdominals hollowed and lifted, and take care not to curve the spine too much. Keep your hips on the floor. Do not sink in to your neck, but lengthen up through your spine. Watch for tension in the neck. If you feel a pinch in your lower back, ease out of the stretch.

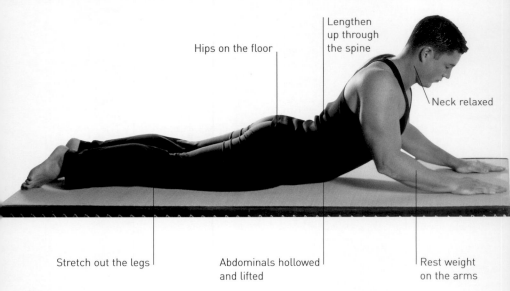

Hips on the floor

Lengthen up through the spine

Neck relaxed

Stretch out the legs

Abdominals hollowed and lifted

Rest weight on the arms

Purpose
To stretch the abdominals.

Target muscles
Abdominals.

Repetitions
Stretch twice; hold for 30 seconds each.

Benefits
- A very good stretch for the abdominals after sport or a workout.
- Targets the main abdominal muscles.
- As well as stretching, you will lengthen the spine.
- Your range of movement will readjust so that you have more freedom and mobility in your daily tasks.
- Regular stretching is linked to a reduced risk of injury.
- After stretching, most people experience a distinct improvement in mood, feeling more refreshed and with a sense of wellbeing.

Checkpoints
- Do not curve your spine too much.
- Keep your head in line with your spine; don't throw your head backward during this stretch.
- Keep facing the floor and lengthen up through the top of your head to avoid your neck sinking in to the shoulders.
- Lift your upper body from the floor as you exhale.
- Watch out for tension in the neck and try to relax your neck and shoulders as much as you can.
- If you feel any pinching in your lower back, ease gently out of the stretch.
- The abdominal muscles should remain hollowed and lifted throughout the stretch, and do not curve the spine too much.
- Keep your hips on the floor.
- Your fingertips should face forward.
- Glide your shoulder blades down your spine.
- If you feel uncomfortable or stiff anywhere in the body, just relax for a while, then try again, taking care not to strain your back or neck.

Hip Flexor Stretch

The hip flexors tend to be one of the tightest muscle groups, and when these muscles get too tight they can cause discomfort and imbalances. People involved in most sports benefit from this stretch, especially runners.

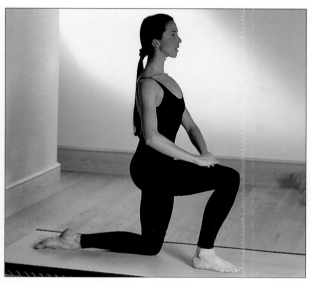

1 Kneel down on the floor and take one step forward, using your hands for support. If you need extra cushioning, place a pillow under the supporting knee.

Focus
- Balance before moving carefully forward in a controlled way; lunge in to the stretch rather than collapse in to it.
- Keep your head facing forward and in alignment throughout the movement.

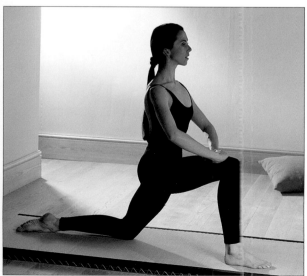

2 Lunge carefully in to the front leg, exhaling as you lunge forward. Make sure your raised knee is directly over your foot. Lengthen up through the spine and keep the abdominals hollowed. You should feel this stretch at the top of the rear leg. Change legs and repeat.

STRETCHES

Purpose
To stretch the hip flexors.

Target muscles
Hip flexors.

Repetitions
Stretch twice; hold for 30 seconds each.

Checkpoints
- Take care not to collapse in to the stretch.
- Lunge in to the stretch.
- Keep your head in alignment.

Benefits
- The tight hip flexors are stretched.
- Works the muscles around the hips.
- People who play sports will benefit from this stretch, especially runners.
- Helps improve posture.
- Good for balance.
- You will feel invigorated after doing this hip flexor stretch.
- Helps to increase your range of movement.

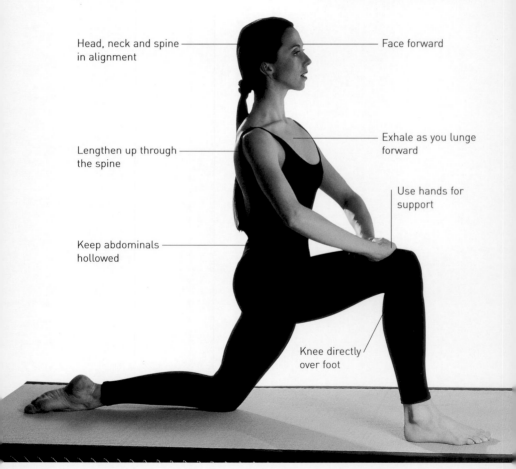

Head, neck and spine in alignment

Face forward

Lengthen up through the spine

Exhale as you lunge forward

Use hands for support

Keep abdominals hollowed

Knee directly over foot

Waist Lifts

This is a good movement to stretch and mobilize the spine. If it feels too intense or uncomfortable to have your arms overhead, then try the stretch with them by your side.

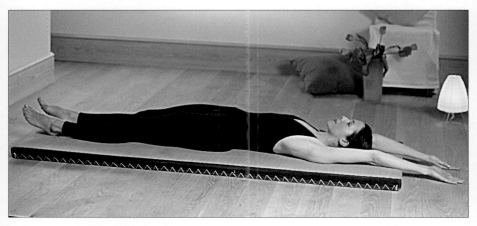

1 Lie on your back with your arms overhead or, if this is difficult, by your sides. Lengthen through your feet, spine and arms: visualize two cars pulling you in different directions. Draw the navel in to the spine.

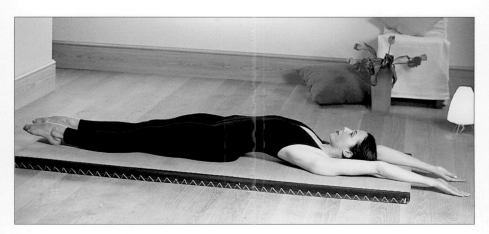

2 Carefully lift your waist. This is a very subtle movement; take care not to create a big curve in your spine. Keep the abdominals strong and the head in alignment. Watch for any gripping in your lower back. If you feel any pinching in your back, ease out of the stretch.

STRETCHES

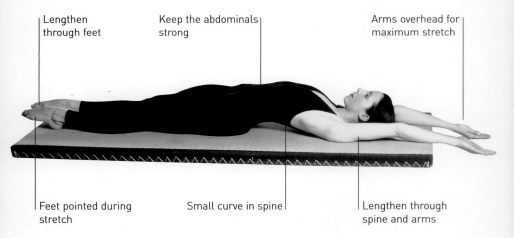

Lengthen through feet

Keep the abdominals strong

Arms overhead for maximum stretch

Feet pointed during stretch

Small curve in spine

Lengthen through spine and arms

Purpose
To stretch and mobilize the spine and reduce any feeling of restriction along the entire spine.

Target muscles
Erector spinae.

Repetitions
Carry out each stretch twice; hold for 30 seconds.

Benefits
- The movement has the effect of stretching out and mobilizing the spine.
- Works the erector spinae muscles.
- As with all stretches, this will improve and lift the mood, inducing a feeling of refreshment and wellbeing.
- Regular practice will give more freedom and mobility and a better range of movement.
- It has been noticed that daily stretching increases flexiblity and causes a reduced rate of injury.

Checkpoints
- Ease out of the stretch if any pinching occurs.
- Keep the abdominals strong.
- Lengthen through your feet, spine and arms by visualizing two forces pulling you in different directions.
- Draw the navel in toward the spine.
- If it feels uncomfortable or too intense to have your arms overhead, then stretch them down by your sides.
- When you lift your waist, do it slowly and purposefully; it is a subtle, rather than a fast, movement.
- Take care not to create too big a curve in your spine.
- Keep the abdominals strong and the head in alignment.
- Watch out for any gripping in your lower back.
- If your back feels uncomfortable during the movement, bring the arms to your sides, ease out of the stretch, and relax.
- Carry out the movements slowly and carefully, without any straining or forcing the body in to uncomfortable positions.
- Watch out for any tension and make a concerted effort to relax completely in to the movement.

Side Stretch

This feels good at any time and can refresh a tired body. No wonder cats and dogs are always stretching – the stretch relieves the body of unwanted tension and liberates the spine and joints.

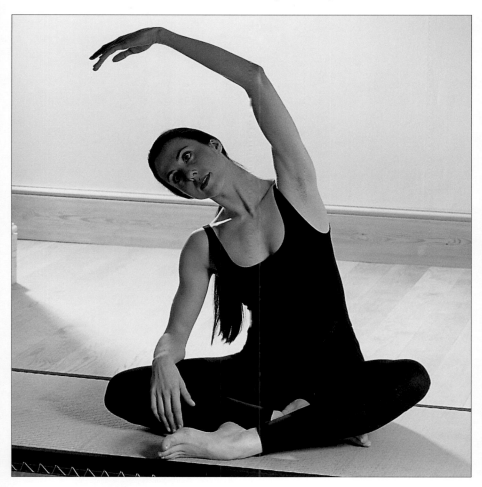

Sit on the floor with one leg in front of the other (the legs are not crossed). Inhale as you prepare. Exhale as you raise one arm and lengthen up through the spine, then stretch in to one side from a strong centre, taking care not to collapse in to the stretch. Feel the stretch in your back. Pull the navel to the spine and keep your buttocks on the floor. If this leg positioning is uncomfortable, instead, bend your legs and keep your feet flat on the floor.

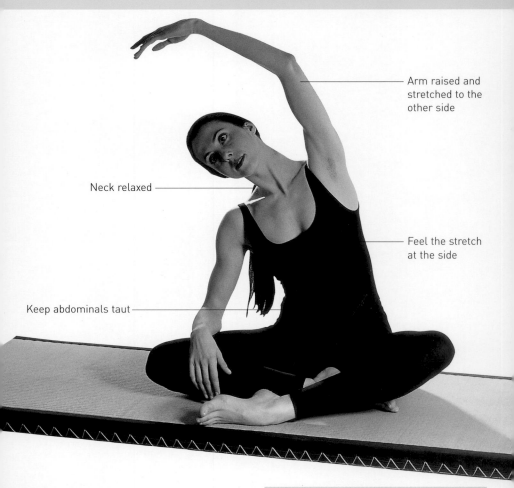

Arm raised and stretched to the other side

Neck relaxed

Feel the stretch at the side

Keep abdominals taut

Purpose
To stretch the back.

Target muscles
The latissimus dorsi.

Repetitions
Stretch twice on each side; hold for 30 seconds each.

Checkpoints
• Keep your buttocks on the floor.
• Lengthen up through the spine.

Benefits
• This stretch relieves the body of unwanted tension.
• Liberates the spine and joints.
• Stretches out the back.
• Targets the latissimus dorsi (muscles in the upper back).
• Because the abdominals are hollowed, this movement helps to create a strong core.
• Produces a feeling of wellbeing.

Basic Back Bend

In this bend, the aim is to lengthen your lower spine down between the buttocks. All you need to do then is lengthen the rest of the spine on top of the hips and you will find achieve a back bend without having bent your back.

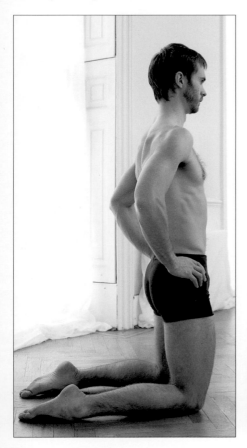

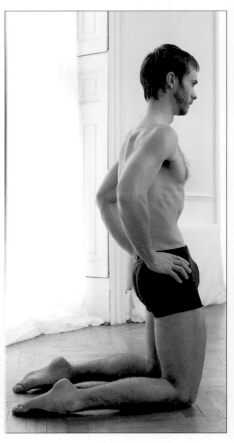

1 Begin in a kneeling position, with the knees positioned directly under your hips. The feeling that you need to achieve is one of lifting the pubic bone with your stomach muscles. If this is difficult at first, simply pull the abdominal muscles in and up. Rest your hands on your hips.

2 Suck in your stomach muscles to try to lift the pubic bone up and through your thighs while you lift and extend your spine. This should keep your tummy tight and trim, and when you recognize that feeling, you can be sure that your spine is protected and lengthened.

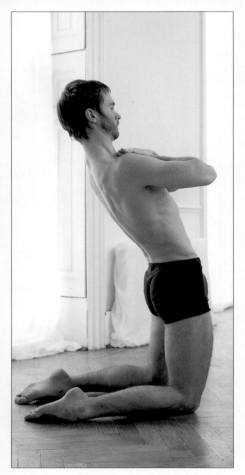

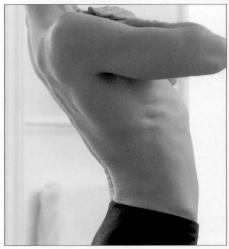

Incorrect
If you do not lift your pubic bone and simply lean backward you will find that the back will bend a lot but you will only move backward a little.

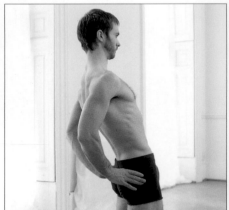

3 Place both hands on your upper chest and push your hands up with your body. Keep the back of your neck long. Do not stop the lift in your tummy and pubic bone. The chest should feel as though it is moving forward and upward, rather than downward and backward. If you feel pressure or discomfort in your lower spine or it feels as if your lower back is doing all the work, go back to opening up the front of your hips and thighs, as this is still limiting the extension of your lower back.

Alternative If you find the back bend difficult, use your hands to help. Push your thumbs in to your sacrum to help hinge the hips up and use your arms to help brace the back out long from the hips. If you feel pain in your lower spine, go back to practising pubic lifts, described in step 1.

Stomach Curl

The pubic lift starts in the stomach. It is easy just to squeeze your bottom to tuck in your tailbone, which provides the same action. Try to achieve the correct action – pressure equally distributed in the body will relieve problems.

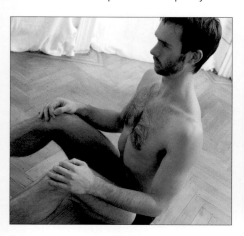

1 Sit with the soles of your feet on the floor and your knees in the air. Sit up as high as you can, pushing down in to the floor. Cup your hands on your knees.

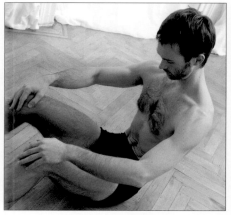

2 As you roll back, point your toes in to the floor and feel your knees push down toward the floor. As you come up, pull your heels toward your buttocks.

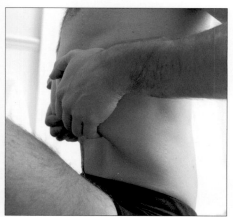

3 With both hands, grab your lower ribs and lift them up. Suck in your stomach and all the muscles that connect from the pubic bone all the way up the front of the body.

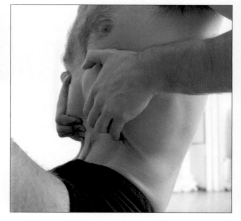

4 As you roll backward, keep lifting your ribs. Your stomach will pull in as before, but now also up in to your rib cage, so you feel a lift in the body as you roll down.

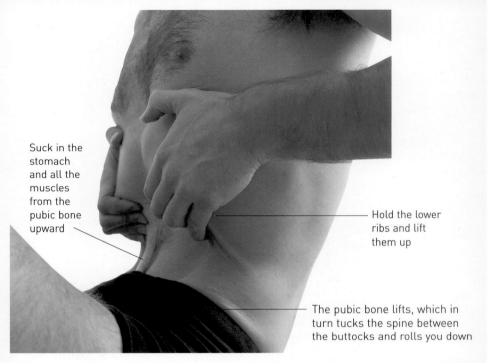

Suck in the stomach and all the muscles from the pubic bone upward

Hold the lower ribs and lift them up

The pubic bone lifts, which in turn tucks the spine between the buttocks and rolls you down

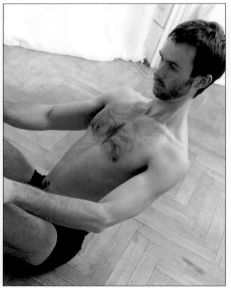

Benefits
- Helps to strengthen the centre of the body; this enables all the other parts to operate more easily.
- Resolves tension in the body and creates balance between the muscles.
- Can help to resolve lower back pain by relieving tension from the hips.

Incorrect (left)
If you simply lean back, rather than roll back, the tummy will bulge. If the arms lengthen before the pubic bone has rolled up, you will know that you have simply leaned back from your chest. This will most probably be accompanied by your abdomen pushing out. The pressure will be in your lower back, not spread evenly in the body, and will cause you problems eventually.

Elbow Lift

In this exercise extend through your legs to your feet. Push your chest high off the floor so you can feel the space between your shoulder blades. The aim of the exercise is to strengthen the stomach muscles.

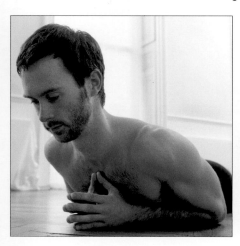

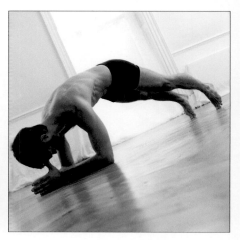

1 Lie on your front and tuck your toes under your heels. Place your hands together, thumbs on your sternum, tucking your elbows in toward your ribs and then push yourself up to balance on your elbows and toes.

2 Lift your pubic bone in to your stomach, as in the Stomach Curl. Practise pulling the abdomen in and up without sticking your bottom out, as that will disengage the stomach muscles, which is the area that this exercise is designed to exercise.

Gravity (right)
You don't have to know about Newtonian mechanics to understand how to use gravity to give you a lift up. See how the hand and the foot both have natural arches, which act like springs pushing up against gravity. Try simply pushing them down and waiting to feel a natural lift in reply.

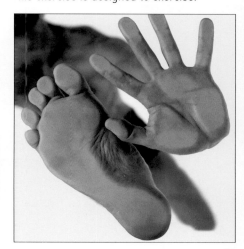

Benefits
- Your stomach muscles will be strengthened and become trained to help to hold you upright.
- Works out the thigh muscles.
- Helps to improve posture and balance.

YOGA-BASED CORE STRENGTH EXERCISES

Alternative

If you find this movement too tricky, rest your knees on the floor, but make sure you really pull your pubic bone up in to your stomach and lengthen the lower spine, or the hip flexors will get a good workout and nothing more.

Incorrect

This shows the classic collapse that usually happens when people try this exercise for the first time. The extremities, especially your toes, take the weight of the body and the lower spine collapses and will soon begin to feel the strain.

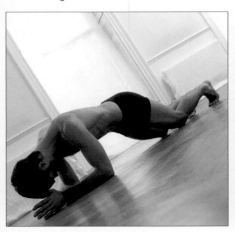

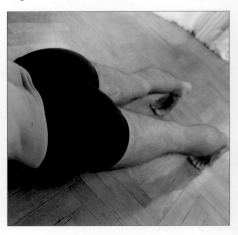

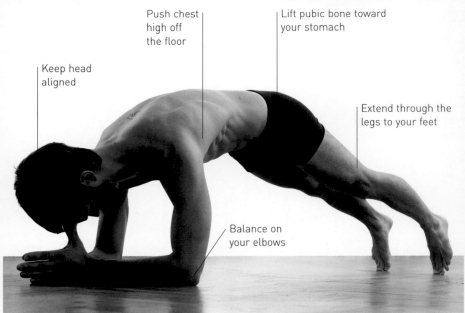

Push chest high off the floor

Lift pubic bone toward your stomach

Keep head aligned

Extend through the legs to your feet

Balance on your elbows

Diamond Curl

This exercise stretches the lower back and loosens the hips. However, if you are doing it properly and rolling from the pubic bone, you will feel the main stretch in the muscles of your legs, especially the hamstrings.

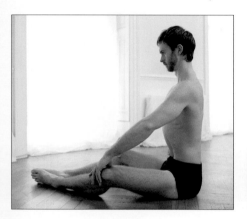 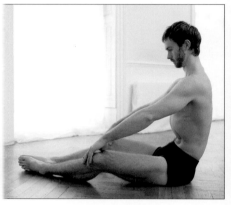

1 Sit on the floor, with your legs in a diamond shape. Sit up as high as you can, pushing your sitting bones down in to the floor. Place your hands firmly on your knees, pushing them down toward the floor. Feel the hip girdle move firmly forward and backward as you roll from the pubic bone.

2 As you roll back, don't be afraid of using your hands. Grab hold of your knees firmly if you need to. Remember to roll your pelvis and feel the movement of the hips between your legs. No matter how flexible you are, there is always room for improvement.

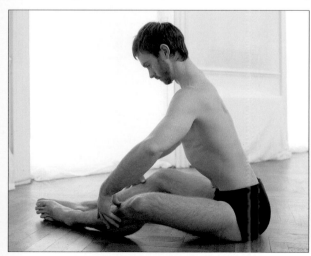

3 Really lean forward, using your hips as a hinge, and you will feel a tug in your hamstrings, the backs of your legs and the inner thighs, as you roll the hips up and over your legs.

Focus
When carried out correctly, the main stretch is in the leg muscles, especially the hamstrings, which stretch down the back of the thigh.

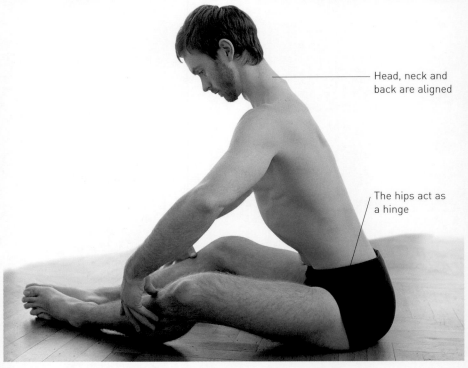

Head, neck and back are aligned

The hips act as a hinge

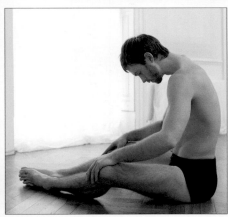

Incorrect
Leading with your head rather than moving your hips forward will not exercise your lower back or stretch your leg muscles.

Benefits
• The lower back is exercised and the hip flexors are loosened. They tend to be one of the tightest muscle groups and can cause discomfort and imbalances, so any exercise that loosens them is beneficial in many ways.
• The leg muscles will be stretched, particularly the hamstring muscles at the back of the thigh.
• Creates a certain level of openness and flexibility in the hip joints. This in turn assists both the range of movement and the flow of energy.
• Loosening the hip flexors helps to reverse a tight lower back and weak abdominal muscles.

Exercise Groups

The following lists will help you to choose a selection of movements from each group to make up a suitable programme. Exercises listed under more than one heading involve a combination of various actions.

Exercises that strengthen the upper body

- Push ups (deltoids, pectorals, biceps, abdominals and stabilizing back muscles)*
- Tricep push-ups (triceps, deltoids, abdominals and pectoral muscles)
- Leg pull prone (abdominals, stabilizing back muscles)*
- Tricep dips (triceps, abdominals)

Exercises that strengthen the lower body

- Cleaning the floor (quadriceps, supporting muscles of the feet and ankles, abdominals)
- The shoulder bridge (buttocks and abdominals)*
- The open V (adductors, abdominals, hip flexors and stabilizing back muscles)
- The outer thigh blaster (abductors, abdominals, adductors and hamstrings)
- One leg kick (hamstrings, abdominals, lower gluteals and erector spinae)*
- The inner thigh lift (adductors, abdominals)

Exercises that strengthen the abdominals and back

- One leg stretch (abdominals and stabilizing back muscles)*
- The side-kick (hamstrings, hip flexors, abdominals, abductors and stabilizing back muscles)*
- The leg pull prone (abdominals and stabilizing back muscles)*
- The roll-up (abdominals and hip flexors)*
- The side bend (obliques, abdominals,

stabilizing back muscles; stretches the latissimus dorsi)*
- One leg circles (adductors, abdominals and hip flexors)*
- The side-squeeze (internal and external obliques, abdominals, shoulder stabilizers and abductors)
- The hundred (abdominals and stabilizing mid-back muscles)*
- The swimming (abdominals, gluteals and erector spinae)*

Exercises that promote flexibility

- Gluteals stretch (gluteals)
- Chest stretch (pectorals)
- Side stretch (latissimus dorsi)
- Hip flexor stretch (hip flexors)
- Spine twist (obliques, adductors and hamstrings; for thoracic mobility)*
- Abdominal stretch (abdominals)
- Spine stretch (erector spinae, hamstrings, adductors)*
- Deep chest and back stretch (pectorals and latissimus dorsi)
- Lower back stretch (erector spinae and gluteals)
- Spine press (erector spinae)

Exercises that promote mobility

- The shoulder bridge (spine)*
- Rolling back (spine)*
- Spine twist (spine)* and Spine press (spine)*
- Spine stretch (spine)*
- One leg circles (hips)*
- Rolling down the spine (spine)*

Core exercises have been marked with an asterisk (*)

Your Pilates Fitness Plan

To work out a suitable plan, you need to assess some factors such as how much time you have to devote to exercising, and what you want to achieve from the movements. The following programmes will help you decide.

In general, Pilates movements can be divided into three main categories:
Strengthening exercises that concentrate on making certain muscle groups stronger and more toned.
Flexibility exercises that improve the range of motion around a joint.
Mobility exercises that train the body to move more easily.

Classifying the movements

The exercises are grouped according to the action that is being reinforced and the muscles used. The following lists repeat this classification to help you choose a selection of movements from each group to make up your programme. If you find an exercise listed under more than one heading it is because it involves a combination of actions.

Core exercises

Your body will need a few sessions to adapt to the movements. Choose a few 'core' exercises and concentrate on these for four to six weeks. Once you feel comfortable and confident about the movements, add more. Try to keep a balance between the main muscles being used: choose one from each group in turn until you have tried them all.

Planning your exercise programme

How much time do you need to dedicate to your Pilates programme? How can you design a programme that will be well-rounded and complete, as well as motivating and enjoyable? When should you change the programme? What if you don't always have time to do it all? To answer these questions you need to take several factors into account.

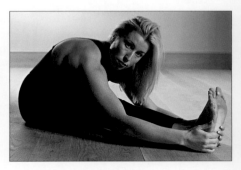

Flexibility exercises will increase your range of movements and help to prevent sports injuries.

1 The time factor

Ideally, you would dedicate at least 1 hour to your Pilates programme and 30–40 minutes to a cardiovascular workout, three times a week. However, if there is no time for a complete training session, a 25-minute workout is better than none.

2 Desired results

Do you want to win a sporting event or just get a little fitter? Dramatic results require dedication, time and effort. But an hour of Pilates three times or even twice a week, as well as three weekly cardiovascular workouts of 30–60 minutes duration, will raise your fitness level in a short time.

3 Daily life

Do you have an active job? Do you live at the top of several flights of stairs? Do you drive everywhere or walk? The things that you do when you are not working out also count. The more sedentary your daily life, the more conscientiously you will have to carry out your fitness plan.

Sample Programme 1

To be effective, exercises need to be organized in to a programme that is easy to remember and that you will want to do regularly. Use this short programme when you are pushed for time but revert to the longer version when you can.

What if you just do not have time to fit in a Pilates session lasting a whole hour? Instead, you can plan a mini programme lasting only 25 minutes to do on those days when you just cannot find more time. However, do try to base most of your sessions around the hour-long plan and use the short programme only when you really have to. Twenty-five minutes is not ideal, but it's better than skipping the session entirely and does bring some benefits. Obviously, you will have to shorten the length of time that you spend on each exercise, as well as doing fewer of them: however, do aim to achieve at least five to seven repetitions of each movement.

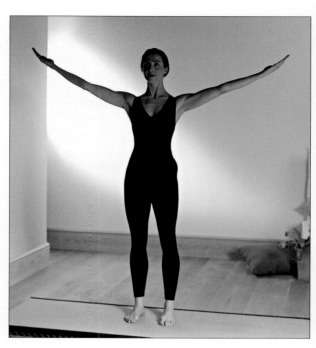

1 Warm-up 8–10 minutes

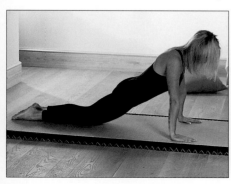

2 Push ups 3 minutes

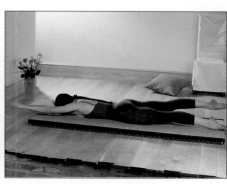

3 The Swimming 3 minutes

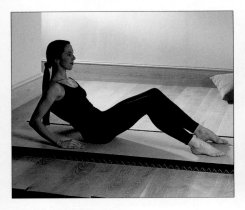

4 Rolling Back 3 minutes

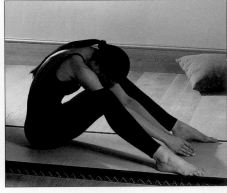

5 Spine Stretch 3 minutes

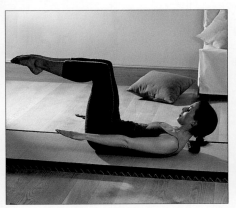

6 The Hundred 3 minutes

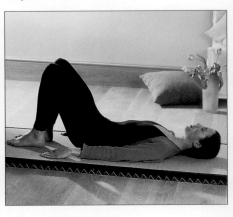

7 Relaxation 2 minutes

Using the short programme

The majority of the exercises need to be repeated approximately ten times each (or, in the case of unilateral exercises, ten times per side).

Apart from one exception – the Hundred is performed for one hundred taps on the mat – when putting together a programme, you can safely estimate that each movement will take about 5 minutes. A certain group of muscles may need more attention because of, for example, muscular imbalances or repetition of a certain activity. You also need to take in to account the initial warm-up, final stretch and a short relaxation period at the end.

Vary your programme from time to time so that you do not get bored. If you dislike an exercise or it does not feel right on a particular day, do a different movement that targets the same muscle groups. Always listen to your body. Most of the exercises have variations, so work your way progressively through the different levels of intensity.

Sample Programme 2

Use this one-hour programme whenever you can to integrate Pilates in to your daily life. Combine a balanced programme with cardiovascular work and good nutrition to give you a total fitness plan.

In this sample format for a one-hour programme, the exercises chosen include some of the 'core' movements; this would be a good programme to start with while you are adapting to the exercises.

As with most Pilates programmes, the emphasis is on the strengthening of the torso. After a few weeks, you can change some of these movements for others; try always to do some movements from each of the different categories so that you are working on all parts of the body and developing strength, flexibility and mobility.

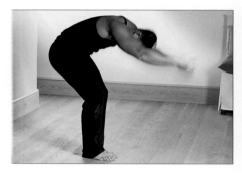

1 Warm-up 8–10 minutes

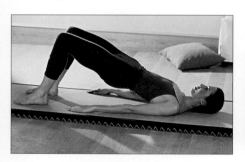

2 The Shoulder Bridge 5 minutes

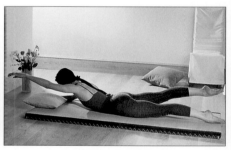

3 The Swimming 5 minutes

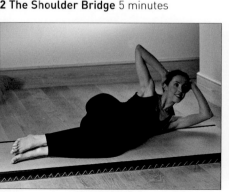

4 Side Squeeze: right side 5 minutes

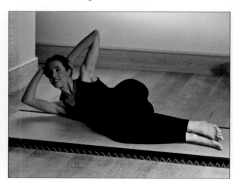

5 Side Squeeze: left side 5 minutes

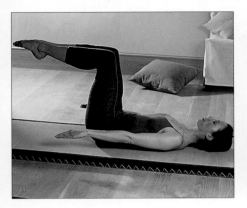

6 The Hundred 5 minutes

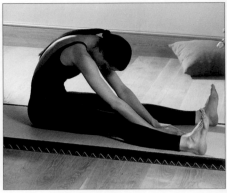

7 Spine Stretch 5 minutes

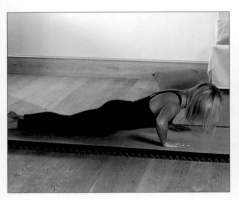

8 Push ups 5 minutes

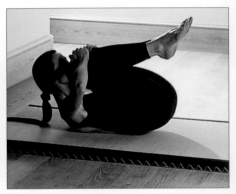

9 Rolling Back 5 minutes

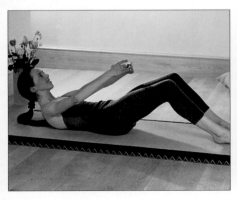

10 The Roll-up 5 minutes

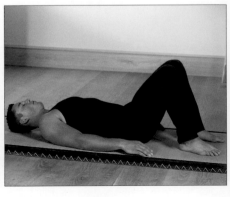

11 Relaxation 5 minutes

Frequently Asked Questions

Regular Pilates practice will improve both your alignment and your posture. Before starting a course, read through these FAQs and check with your doctor that it is appropriate exercise for your state of health.

Will Pilates help me lose weight?
Losing weight – or rather fat – is a question of disrupting the energy balance, between calories in and calories out. A regular exercise programme will raise the body's metabolism, and although the amount of calories burnt per session may be quite small, over a period of time they will add up. Pilates, combined with a cardiovascular programme and a sensible diet, will give you the results you desire.

I would like to start exercising again but last time I went to the gym I just got bulky. I really dislike the current trend to be very muscular; can Pilates help?
Yes it can. Pilates builds long, lean muscles by keeping repetitions and resistance low. As it pays special attention to alignment, every move is designed to elongate as it strengthens, which is ideal for anyone who builds bulk easily.

When will I start to see results? I cannot seem to stick to any programme long enough to see any real benefits.
If you combine Pilates about three times a week with a cardiovascular programme and a sound diet, you should see visible results within four weeks. Your arms and legs will start to look more toned. Your back will be stronger and your tummy may look flatter. However, the change won't only be visible. You will notice positive changes within yourself. You will start looking forward to your workouts and feel stronger. You will sleep better and will most probably be in a better mood. Your aerobic sessions will become easier and you will be able to exercise for longer periods at a time. Give it a try for a month: it's worth it.

I have quite a sway back (lordosis) and frequently experience back pain just above the kidneys. Will Pilates aggravate this?
Anyone with an injury or back problem should seek medical advice before starting this or any exercise programme. Pilates is an excellent technique for correcting certain postural deviations and strengthening weaknesses. However, it should not be used as a remedial method unless it is supervised by a trained and certified professional. Pilates will aggravate a situation such as lordosis if the movements are improperly executed.

I play golf every weekend and find that I often suffer from a stiff back and neck after a game. Which exercises would be helpful in relieving or preventing this?
Pilates is an excellent training method for golfers as the customary action in this sport is quite often a hazardous one for the back. You should follow the whole programme, as all the movements will be beneficial. You may be pleasantly surprised as you discover that your game is improving with your improved strength and flexibility.

I have never exercised at all but would like to start with this programme. Could this be dangerous? I am a 54-year-old woman, slightly overweight and a non-smoker.
You should seek medical advice before starting this or any other exercise programme if you have any injuries or risk factors. These would include coronary heart disease, diabetes, high blood pressure, high cholesterol, obesity, a heavy smoking habit or a very sedentary lifestyle. Women over 50 and sedentary men over 40 should also check with their doctors.

GLOSSARY

Breathe laterally Breathe wide and full in to the ribs, taking them out to the sides as you inhale and bringing them back together as you exhale. Avoid breathing in to the stomach or high in to the chest.

Core strength This term is given to the muscles of the torso which control all core movements in Pilates.

Control Work within a range of movements that you can control. Do not use momentum to increase the range; it will not work your muscles to the same extent.

Feet flexed This is the opposite of pointing your toes. Pull your toes back to the shin bone.

Flow All Pilates movements should be smooth and continuous. To help maintain flow, imagine moving through soft mud.

Glide the shoulder blades down the spine Avoid hunching the shoulders. Practise by first hunching your shoulders up to your ears and then slide them back down your spine to reduce tension at the neck and shoulders.

Gripping Gripping is the unnecessary overuse of the muscles, especially around the neck, hip flexors, feet, shoulders and lower back. It creates tension in the muscles.

Hollow out the abdominals Imagine pulling the navel toward your spine, as if you were wearing tight trousers and want to create space between the waistband and your tummy by using the abdominals.

Lengthening Imagine a balloon positioned in the centre of your head. Picture it floating up to the ceiling and try to create space between each vertebra in your spine.

Neutral spine To check if your spine is in the correct, natural position, flatten your back to the floor then arch it. Neutral spine is the comfortable position between the two. This position protects your spine.

Ribs flaring up The ribs should travel out to the sides as you breathe. Maintain the distance between the hips and ribs rather than letting the ribs travel up toward the chest as this involves arching the spine.

Tilt the pelvis This simply means pointing the pubic bone up toward your chin.

ACKNOWLEDGEMENTS

This edition is published by Lorenz Books, an imprint of Anness Publishing Ltd, Blaby Road, Wigston, Leicestershire LE18 4SE; info@anness.com

www.lorenzbooks.com; www.annesspublishing.com

If you like the images in this book and would like to investigate using them for publishing, promotions or advertising, please visit our website www.practicalpictures.com for more information.

A CIP catalogue record for this book is available from the British Library

Publisher: Joanna Lorenz
Editor: Anne Hildyard
Photography: Clare Park, Christine Hanscomb, Stephen Swain, John Freeman
Models: Kelda Dearden, Kelvin Everitt, Emily Kelly, Jonathan Monks

PUBLISHER'S NOTE
The author and publishers have made every effort to ensure that all instructions contained within this book are accurate and safe, and cannot accept liability for any resulting injury, damage or loss to persons or property, however it may arise. If you do have any special needs or problems, consult your doctor or another health professional. This book cannot replace medical consultation and should be used in conjunction with professional advice. You should not attempt Pilates without training from a properly qualified practitioner.

Material previously published as part of a larger book: *Pilates and Yoga*.